Praise for

INCURABLE FAITH

"Most people either resist or resent pain, but Andrea Herzer has harnessed it to forge a path of unparalleled wisdom and compassion. If you or a loved one are dealing with the pain of illness, *Incurable Faith* is a significant contribution of sustenance, blessing, and inspiration to equip you for the journey."

> —JOHN C. MAXWELL, author, speaker, and leadership expert

"In the midst of her own physical hardships, Andrea has created a book that will help you discover intimacy with God, find unexplainable joy, and develop a deep stabilizing faith."

> —CHRYSTAL EVANS HURST, co-host of *The Sister Circle Podcast*
> and co-author of *Divine Disruption*

"Andrea Herzer has a heart for those who suffer because she's lived it. *Incurable Faith* is a gift to anyone who is suffering and is longing to taste the goodness of God in the desolate places of their lives."

> —VANEETHA RENDALL RISNER, author of *The Scars That Have Shaped Me*

"*Incurable Faith* is a book that should be in the hands of anyone suffering from a chronic illness or caring for someone who is chronically ill. Every aspect of this book takes you deep into the heart of our Lord Jesus."

> —JANE DALY, author of *The Caregiving Season*

"Andrea Herzer intertwines her heart for the suffering with her faith in Christ to offer a cool cup of water to the hurting. Read this book slowly, be encouraged, and revel in the living hope to which Herzer points."

> —KATHRYN BUTLER, MD, trauma surgeon and author of
> *Between Life and Death*

"Anyone who is facing a brutal diagnosis, being crushed by pain, or being sidelined by what she did not choose is going to find hope and life in these pages."

—MARGOT STARBUCK, author of *Small Things with Great Love*

"I encourage anyone who has had health challenges, life-altering diagnoses, and heart-wrenching outcomes, to take the journey with Andrea as she navigates the unknown with her *Incurable Faith* in God."

—KIMBERLEE SULLIVAN, board-certified clinical specialist in women's health physical therapy

"Andrea's style of reflecting about who God is and how His Word speaks to us amid pain, trials, and difficulty has a raw beauty. *Incurable Faith* will restore the hope in your life that you may have lost along the way."

—TIM HAWKS, lead pastor of Hill Country Bible Church Austin

"If you're facing a serious health issue yourself—or if you're a loved one, caregiver, or provider who wants to better understand and process these challenging times—Andrea's book is a steady guide and faithful companion that will show you how to pray, embrace, ponder, and worship through whatever you're facing."

—W. LEE WARREN, MD, neurosurgeon and award-winning author of *I've Seen the End of You*

"*Incurable Faith* is the gift you've been looking for when you don't know what to say or how to reach out to someone who has an insurmountable health crisis."

—CAROL KENT, speaker and bestselling author of *When I Lay My Isaac Down*

"When the unwelcome, unwanted, and unbelievably difficult comes knocking at your door, open the pages of this book and let *Incurable Faith* usher hope and help into your home and heart."

—PAM FARREL, bestselling co-author of *Discovering Hope in the Psalms*

INCURABLE FAITH

INCURABLE
FAITH

120 Devotions of Lasting Hope

for Lingering Health Issues

ANDREA HERZER

Multnomah

Published in the United States by Multnomah, an imprint of Random House, a division of Penguin Random House LLC.

MULTNOMAH is a registered trademark and the M colophon is a trademark of Penguin Random House LLC.

The Cataloging-in-Publication Data is on file with the Library of Congress.

Printed in the United States of America on acid-free paper

waterbrookmultnomah.com

1st Printing

First Edition

Interior book design by Virginia Norey
Abstract background art by: sokolart/stock.adobe.com

SPECIAL SALES Most Multnomah books are available at special quantity discounts when purchased in bulk by corporations, organizations, and special-interest groups. Custom imprinting or excerpting can also be done to fit special needs. For information, please email specialmarketscms@penguinrandomhouse.com.

To Jesus, my savior, who has been "a shelter from the storm and a shade from the heat" (Isaiah 25:4)

And to my husband, Mark, who joined me in the storm, carried the umbrella, and never left my side

CONTENTS

SECTION ONE:

A Satisfying Snack

SECTION TWO:

A Marvelous Meal

SECTION THREE:

A Fabulous Feast

A Letter from
My Heart to Yours

Beloved reader,

I'm glad you're here, because I wrote this book for you. If you are living with health challenges or are a support person for someone who is, *Incurable Faith* is for you. If you're the person who smiles through the pain while facing treatments, surgeries, and uncertainties that no one else seems to understand, *Incurable Faith* holds hope for you. If you're the person who fears disease progression or disability, these words will encourage you. If you're the person fighting hard to hold on to life or even battling the urge to give up, *Incurable Faith* will strengthen you. If you're the caregiver, medical provider, family member, or friend who supports those afflicted by health issues, this book will equip you to persevere with greater compassion.

Living with health challenges can create a deep sense of loneliness during a time when you need people the most. Even supportive loved ones might not understand the depths of your pain, fear, and sadness about your medical issues. If you're desperately trying to find a diagnosis for your baffling symptoms, you might even begin to question your ability to trust your own feelings. You may feel the grief of shattered dreams, and even shattered friendships, when health issues limit your activities or confine you to home or a hospital. How do I know about these thoughts and feelings? I've experienced them all and more, having lived with life-altering health issues for over two decades. In fact, when I began writing these devotions, I had no idea my future would hold more than one hundred medical procedures, increasing disability, and aggressive advanced-stage cancer.

As the daughter of a physician, I grew up hearing about the ravages of illness from a doctor's perspective. But my experiences with decades of debilitating illness have taught me the true burdens and secret worries of a patient. In *Incurable Faith,* you will read about my private struggles and learn how Jesus has met me and continues to meet me in my pain. You will discover His sufficiency in every sorrow and find His peace for every worry. You will learn the practices that will fill you with overflowing joy despite any diagnosis. These are just a few of the Scripture-based and life-tested truths I have brought together in *Incurable Faith.*

When I began my own journey with life-altering health issues, I wanted a guidebook that would show me how to live well while feeling unwell. I found books about suffering and books by those who had already been healed. But there were few inspirational Christian books by authors with ongoing medical issues, written *during* their health challenges.

I had been a follower of Jesus for many years, even working in ministry, but I wasn't fully prepared to undergo this depth of suffering. My faith was being refined and tested, but I secretly began to wonder if God was punishing me. Didn't Jesus promise abundant life to His followers?

I was hungry for healing, but God satisfied my hunger with an unexpected feast. He provided wisdom for my walk, mercy for my mess, and hope for my heart. Almost seven years after my first diagnosis, I began to chronicle my daily health battles by sharing how Scripture helped me fight. I dreamed that these devotions would one day bring hope to others who suffer from medical issues.

What I *never* dreamed was that my journey through illness was far from over. But I am a living testimony that you can embrace a beautifully abundant life even during a devastating diagnosis.

So curl up and settle into a cozy space. Snuggle into a blanket and tuck into comfort as you read the following devotions. Get ready to live *with* your health issues by living *within* infectious joy and incurable faith.

With love and blessings,

Andrea

A Note About
the Format and Content

Reading a book or studying the Bible can seem overwhelming when you have health issues. Medical treatments, medication side effects, and chronic illnesses often limit attention span and concentration. I understand these limitations, so I grouped the devotions by length instead of by topic. But I also included a topical index in the back of the book. You can choose what to read based on your need each day, or you can read the book from cover to cover!

How to decide what to read each day:

- *Do you have a specific need, such as perseverance, hope, or strength?*

    The **topical index** on pages 273–277 will help you find a devotion.

- *Do your health issues impair your ability to focus on a lengthy devotion?*

    Section One: A Satisfying Snack offers short messages that are meant to replenish and revive your spirit when health issues limit concentration and attention span.

- *Do you feel well enough to sink into a heartier devotion?*

    Section Two: A Marvelous Meal has medium-length entries that are just right for days when you have the energy and ability to focus on reading a slightly longer passage.

- *Do you want the comfort of spending some extended time in Scripture?*

Section Three: A Fabulous Feast contains the longest devotions. Each stand-alone chapter might be just the right choice when you are lonely and want the extra comfort of a lengthier quiet time.

Each devotion includes these components:

- **Scripture**—a verse to plant in your heart and mind
- **Passage**—a devotion to help you through life with health issues
- **Prayer**—a short conversation with God
- **Truth to Embrace**—a concise takeaway truth to embrace throughout the day
- **Worship Song**—music to accompany the day's devotion, with a Spotify playlist of all the songs available at www.andreaherzer.com/playlist.

Sections Two and Three include one of the following:

- **Ponder**—how the passage relates to your own life
- **Practice**—an action that will enrich your faith and your life

I understand the burdens of illness, so I wrote *Incurable Faith* with your needs in mind. There are no dates on devotions because I know how hard it can be to keep up with a daily format when you have surgeries or treatments. The scripture is written out to make it easily accessible, but I encourage you to open your Bible or Bible app and read the entire passage. You may also choose to keep a journal and pen or a voice-assisted computer nearby to record your Ponder answers and complete your Practice exercises. I chose not to include an area to record your responses in the book so as not to discourage those who are unable to use writing utensils. However you choose to respond—whether by voice-assisted technology, typing, or handwriting—recording your thoughts after reading a passage can be a helpful practice and a wonderful way to later reflect on your journey.

Last, you won't want to miss the Resources section (beginning on page 261), which is full of helpful information. There you will find encouraging scriptures and books for further reading, as well as crisis-hotline numbers and even a twenty-four-hour prayer line. Caregivers will find recommended books and websites to assist and support them.

I pray that as you read *Incurable Faith*, you will experience the powerful presence of God and know beyond a shadow of a doubt that you are not alone and are dearly loved.

Spotify playlist of recommended worship songs:
www.andreaherzer.com/playlist

A Satisfying Snack

This section offers short messages to replenish and revive your spirit when health issues limit concentration and attention span.

He satisfies the longing soul,

and *the hungry soul* he fills

with GOOD things.

—Psalm 107:9, ESV

The Proper Place

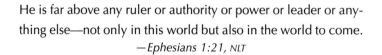

He is far above any ruler or authority or power or leader or anything else—not only in this world but also in the world to come.
—Ephesians 1:21, NLT

No doctor ever proclaimed, "You have cancer," when I was diagnosed with non-Hodgkin lymphoma. My father, a physician,
responded to a texted photo of my bulging neck by texting back, "It
looks like lymphoma," so I knew cancer was a possibility. My primary-
care doctor said, "Your CT scan is suspicious for lymphoma." My
surgeon told me the specific types of lymphoma revealed in my biopsy. Although no one uttered the words *You have cancer,* the words *I
have cancer* filled my mind for weeks.

You have likely felt dread in the pit of your stomach upon hearing
bad news. That is how I felt whenever I thought, *I have cancer.* But
Jesus is more powerful than any disease. Even cancer. The thought
that I had cancer took my breath away, so I inhaled peace by replac-
ing that thought with this one: *I have Jesus.* The power of that beautiful name restores me. Cancer stays in its proper place when I place
my trust in Jesus. Today I still have cancer, but one day I will have
eternal healing from every disease—and I will still have Jesus.

Pray: Jesus, Your name is above every other name. You are my
healer, savior, and friend. One day You will rise with healing in
Your wings to destroy the power of every disease. Fill me with
Your Holy Spirit, and give me all I need to endure until that
day. In Your mighty name I pray. Amen.

Embrace: My disease stays in its proper place when I put my trust in Jesus.

Worship: "What a Beautiful Name/Agnus Dei (Medley)" by Travis Cottrell, featuring Lily Cottrell

Trust the Teacher

—╀————————————╀—

I will lead the blind by ways they have not known, along unfamiliar paths I will guide them; I will turn the darkness into light
before them and make the rough places smooth. These are the
things I will do; I will not forsake them.
—*Isaiah 42:16*

I taught a spunky visually impaired student named Kelly in my
first-grade class. Kelly was new to the school, so she depended on
a mobility teacher to help her safely navigate the unfamiliar environment. The teacher took her through the school hallways and gave
instructions along the way. Kelly eventually learned that she could
trust her teacher to guide her to the places she needed to go.

You may feel unsure and lost when illness alters the landscape of
your life. But you are not alone. Jesus is the teacher who guides you.
He does not watch from afar as you navigate the difficulties of illness. He knows the way through your challenges and will take you
safely through every twist and turn. Your confident trust in the Lord
will increase as He guides you; you do not travel through illness
alone.

Pray: Dear God, thank You for guiding me and teaching me to
navigate difficult paths. You made a way for me to have eternal
life, and You make a way through everything I face. Thank You
for illuminating the steps I need to take to move forward. Keep
my foot from every wrong path; guide me on the way that leads
to life. In Jesus's name, amen.

Embrace: Jesus helps me navigate the difficulties of illness.

Worship: "You Know My Name" by Tasha Cobbs Leonard, featuring Jimi Cravity

Blessed Opportunities

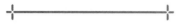

How can they call on him to save them unless they believe in him? And how can they believe in him if they have never heard about him? And how can they hear about him unless someone tells them?

—*Romans 10:14, NLT*

E arlier this week, I called a friend who had just learned her mother has cancer. I prayed with her and shared scriptures that helped me during my own cancer diagnosis. A repairman in my home overheard our conversation, and when I hung up the phone, he told me that two of his family members were also fighting cancer. His heart was heavy for them. Our conversation easily shifted to spiritual matters, so I shared with him the comforts of faith in Christ. I have met many people who are eager to receive spiritual truth when health issues burden them. Illness is hard to bear, but it opens up blessed opportunities to share gospel hope.

Pray: Lord, may my story be an encouragement to others. Let them witness Your power as You turn weakness into strength and trials into blessings. May even the unexpected disappointments in my life serve as a platform to bring glory to You. Give me the courage and opportunity to tell others the good news of Jesus Christ. Amen.

Embrace: My illness can open up opportunities to tell others about Jesus.

Worship: "Each One, Reach One" by Babbie Mason

The Provider Always Provides

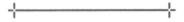

Look at the birds of the air; they do not sow or reap or store away in barns, and yet your heavenly Father feeds them. Are you not much more valuable than they?
—*Matthew 6:26*

God often provides for our needs through other people, but we cannot expect them to meet our every demand during illness. Sometimes we might be overwhelmed by the outpouring of support. Other times we are undone by loneliness and lack. I am humbled when people help me during illness and further humbled when they do not.

When I fully trust God as my provider, I can release others from the burden of meeting the tremendous needs that arise with illness. He often provides in ways I least expect, so I must be open to His plan during this season of my life. I am learning to be flexible and patient. God may be working in the hearts of people around me to teach them how to serve, or He may be training my heart to discern my real needs. Either way, the Provider always supplies what is best.

Pray: Dear God, You are my provider. I will approach Your throne with confidence, and I will approach people with grace and love. When they cannot help me, please enable me to release any offense so that no root of bitterness will grow in my heart. Thank You for all the ways You provide for me. In Jesus's name, amen.

Embrace: God uses great need to develop greater faith.

Worship: "He's Always Been Faithful" by Sara Groves

The Secret Step

I have refined you, though not as silver; I have tested you in the
furnace of affliction.

—*Isaiah 48:10*

Homemade organic chicken broth is a staple in my home. I put
freshly diced vegetables and a whole chicken into a pot with
clear water. Then I add a handful of parsley, savory herbs, and a few
peppercorns. The ingredients are a bouquet of freshness and flavor.
But even the best ingredients will produce a cloudy chicken broth if
I don't take an additional step. The secret to creating a clear broth is
to carefully skim off the foamy gray substance that accumulates on
the simmering surface of the liquid. Could I expect to produce an
appealing broth without removing the impurities? Of course not!
Yet I become just like that unappetizing broth when I stew in indig-
nation, anger, and bitterness about my health issues without the additional cleansing step of repentance. God uses the fires of affliction
to bring my impurities to the surface so that confession and grace
can completely skim them away.

Pray: Dear God, help me remember that stewing in anger or
bitterness will make the fires of affliction feel unbearable.
Chronic illness is a long simmering process; use it to test and
transform me. Refresh me during my heated trials. Your
strength is the ingredient that enables me to endure. Thank You
for loving me enough to make me into a new creation. In Jesus's
name, amen.

Embrace: My afflictions bring impurities to the surface so that confession and grace can completely skim them away.

Worship: "Refiner" by Maverick City Music, featuring Chandler Moore and Steffany Gretzinger

Getting in Shape

Like clay in the hand of the potter, so are you in my hand.
—*Jeremiah 18:6*

My children loved to play with modeling clay when they were young. Their tiny hands pounded it until it was pliable. Then they patted it into various flower or seashell molds that I kept just for that purpose. Sometimes they pressed the clay into a mold and forgot about it. When it dried, it remained in the shape of the mold.

Debilitating illness presses hard; it crushes every last vestige of self-reliance and pride out of us. There are times when suffering is so deep that it changes us completely. We become pliable and ready to be molded, for better or worse, by what we cling to during trials. What do you cling to when you are hard-pressed by illness? Let your ailments press you closer to Jesus so you will be shaped and transformed into His beautiful image.

Pray: Dear God, change me into the person You created me to be. My suffering is reshaping me; I am ready to be molded. Teach me how to press into Jesus so I will be transformed into His image. Help me wholeheartedly cling to You during my trials. Amen.

Embrace: I will cling to Jesus so I can be transformed into His image.

Worship: "Close to You (Live)" by Mosaic MSC

Worst-Case Scenario

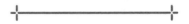

Be not wise in your own eyes; fear the LORD, and turn away from evil. It will be healing to your flesh and refreshment to your bones.

—Proverbs 3:7–8, ESV

I had a unique superpower when my children were small: I could glance into a room and immediately find every safety hazard. The sharp table corners and open outlets were no match for me! That skill may have helped me protect my toddlers, but it hurts me when I apply it to my health issues.

I look into every potential negative outcome when I'm given a new diagnosis. Then I tell myself I'm being realistic by mentally preparing for the worst-case scenario. But the truth is that these ruminations actually arise out of fear and unbelief. When thoughts are filled with trepidation *about* the future, they leave no room to consider God's sufficiency *for* the future.

We want to be realistic when facing illness, but is it reasonable to imagine a future without the presence of an omnipotent God? Our days belong to the God whose thoughts and ways are beyond human comprehension. None of us can accurately predict the future with a mind that is limited to the present. So I will stop my vain imagining, and I will trust the God who is able to do immeasurably more than I can imagine with every aspect of my life.

Pray: Dear God, thank You that my life is in Your hands. I never need to imagine a future apart from Your loving care. Please stop my fearful and worried thoughts. I choose to rest in You; I trust You with my future. In Jesus's name, amen.

Embrace: I will be a realist by embracing the fear-reducing reality that I can trust God with my future.

Worship: "Because He Lives (Amen)" by Matt Maher

Come to My Aid

Contend, LORD, with those who contend with me; fight against those who fight against me. Take up shield and armor; arise and come to my aid.

—Psalm 35:1–2

When I was a child, I had two friends at school who were my constant companions. We were all sweet little girls individually, but something happened when the three of us got together. There is a reason for the saying "Three is a crowd," and it must have been coined by a teacher! Inevitably, two of us would side against one, and tears would ensue. There was usually a teacher nearby watching and waiting to help. Sometimes she separated us to prevent conflict; other times she let us work things out for ourselves. But she always comforted the one who had been hurt.

The psalmist David said, "You have taken from me friend and neighbor—darkness is my closest friend" (Psalm 88:18). Often pain and illness seem like our closest companions. They regularly take sides against us. But we have a teacher named Jesus. Sometimes He shields us from their attacks; other times He assists us in the fight so our faith will grow. But He is there without fail, watching and ready to come to our aid. And He always brings comfort.

Pray: Lord, thank You that You are always by my side. I need You today. Sometimes You separate me from my hardships, and other times You give me what I need to endure them. But You never forsake me. Be my helper today. Be my advocate in my fight with illness. I submit all of myself to You today. I will rest in Your watchful care. In Your precious name I pray. Amen.

Embrace: Jesus is always ready to come to my aid; He assists and comforts me when health issues rise up against me.

Worship: "Always (Live)" by Passion, featuring Kristian Stanfill

Resting on My Foundation

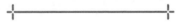

Be still, and know that I am God.
—*Psalm 46:10*

Do you ever feel trapped by the limitations of being in bed with illness? You might long to get up and be active, but your body has other plans. One day I was bemoaning my bedridden state of exhaustion and pain. I sought physical comfort by sinking down into my soft mattress, and the sensation reminded me to sink my thoughts into the comfort of worship. God brings healing contentment to my soul when I meditate on His character instead of the characteristics of my illness.

He is holy. He is just. He is merciful. He is loving. He is sovereign. He is good. He is my provider. He is my healer. He is my friend. God's character cannot be characterized by my limitations. Health issues may temporarily bind us, but His love is boundless. We are lifted above the frustrations of our limitations when we lift up God's name. Peace blankets the bedridden stillness when we rest our thoughts on Him.

Pray: Dear God, there are times when I want anything but stillness in my life. I long to be active and well. Teach me how I can be active in my faith, praise, and prayers when I am inactive because of my health struggles. Help me rest in Your care when I am in bed with illness. When I sink into the comfort of the mattress beneath me, I remember that You are my foundation. I will rest my thoughts on You. In Jesus's name, amen.

Embrace: God brings healing contentment to my soul when I meditate on His character instead of the characteristics of my illness.

Worship: "Be Still My Soul (In You I Rest)" by Kari Jobe

A Reason to Rally

When Jacob was told, "Your son Joseph has come to you," Israel rallied his strength and sat up on the bed.

—*Genesis 48:2*

L iving every day with chronic pain, illness, and fatigue means we have many occasions to summon our strength. Sometimes our love for others propels us beyond ourselves. We get out of bed to take care of family members or visit with friends while everything inside us is screaming for rest. At times, we rally because we are determined to complete tasks the Lord has placed on our hearts. I rally my strength during overwhelming pain and fatigue to write devotionals to bless others just as Jacob rallied his strength to bless his son. We all need a reason to rally. What is yours?

Pray: Dear God, there are days when I cannot rally much strength at all. Give me all I need to get through those days. Propel me by the power of Your Holy Spirit. Fill me with the love and purpose that give me a reason to keep going. I can summon my strength because You are my strength. In Jesus's name, amen.

Embrace: My love for God and others can help me rally my strength every day.

Worship: "Christ Be All Around Me (Live)" by Leeland, featuring All Sons & Daughters

The Laundry Room Song

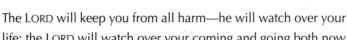

The LORD will keep you from all harm—he will watch over your life; the LORD will watch over your coming and going both now and forevermore.

—Psalm 121:7–8

I helped my three children memorize Bible verses for school by making each verse into a song. We sang the verses throughout the week until they were easy to recall. According to my children, my terrible singing gave them great incentive to learn their scriptures quickly. Once, I wrote out Psalm 121:7–8 on a large whiteboard in our laundry room to help them memorize it. I would softly (okay, loudly at times!) sing it to myself while doing the laundry. Doing laundry exacerbated my pain, so this particular passage reminded me that the Lord watched over me to keep me from actual harm. Placing God's Word in an area of your home where you are most apt to need it can give you the comfort and strength to make it through the day.

Pray: Dear Lord, thank You that Your Word comforts and strengthens me. Prompt me to recall scriptures when pain, brain fog, and fatigue cloud my mind. Please give me the wisdom to plan ahead for those difficult days. Help me hold Your Word in my heart by having it easily accessible in my home. Thank You that it both sustains and saves me. Amen.

Embrace: I will hold God's Word in my heart by making it easily accessible in my home.

Worship: "Your Word" by Christine D'Clario

His Presence Brings Peace

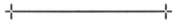

On the evening of that first day of the week, when the disciples
were together, with the doors locked for fear of the Jewish leaders, Jesus came and stood among them and said, "Peace be with
you!"

—John 20:19

In Jesus's first appearance to the disciples after His resurrection,
He greeted them by proclaiming, "Peace be with you!" In the original Greek, the word for "peace" is *eiréné*, which implies complete
wholeness, tranquility, and rest. Jesus entered the room that the disciples' fear had locked, and He gave them the peace they needed.
Their difficult circumstances were the same, but Jesus in their midst
meant that everything had changed. His presence gave them peace
that unlocked their courage and restored their faith. Invite Jesus into
the midst of your health struggles. His presence will always bring
peace.[1]

Pray: Jesus, I need courage and faith right now. I invite You
into the midst of my struggle with pain and illness. Restore me,
Lord. I receive Your complete wholeness, tranquility, and rest
today. Amen.

Embrace: Jesus brings tranquility and peace when I invite
Him into my struggles.

Worship: "Nothing Else" by Cody Carnes

Connected, Not Rejected

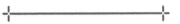

Now you are the body of Christ, and each one of you is a part of it.

—1 Corinthians 12:27

L ong-term health issues can be isolating. They might even prevent you from enjoying the active life you once led. While undergoing surgeries, treatments, or infusions, your only human interaction might be with medical staff. And if you are bedridden or homebound, you already know the brutal isolation that illness imposes. But no matter where your health issues take you or leave you, they can never keep you from your position in the body of Christ. Those who have accepted Jesus Christ are forever part of His body. Illness and fatigue may prevent you from regularly attending church or enjoying an active social life, but they can never keep you from filling the place in the body that only you can fill. You are forever connected, never rejected, and always loved.

Pray: Dear God, there are times when I feel so alone. But the truth is that when I accepted Jesus, I became forever connected to other believers. Thank You that I have a special place in the body of Christ. Illness may isolate me from others at times, but You have loved me enough to make me part of Your forever family. Thank You, Lord. Amen.

Embrace: The isolation of illness cannot separate me from the body of Christ.

Worship: "How Beautiful" by Twila Paris

You Are Radiant

—————————|—————————————————|—————————

Those who look to him are radiant; their faces are never covered with shame.

—*Psalm 34:5*

The first time one of my health issues demanded privacy was when childbirth complications created the need for additional surgeries. I'd presumed that my ob-gyn surgeon's nurse would follow medical privacy laws, so I was unprepared when her husband walked up to me at church and announced, "I hear you had surgery! My wife talks in her sleep." My face grew hot with shame and anger. Although inappropriate, his comment did not create my shame. It merely uncovered this truth: I *already* felt ashamed of my afflictions and even more ashamed of their cures.

Are you undergoing difficult medical treatments to regain your health? You might need pessary devices, drains, or suppositories. You may have lost all your hair or even parts of your body. Do you feel embarrassed by your medical issues? Reflecting on the indignity of illness opens a door for shame to enter. Reflect instead on God's estimation of your unchangeable worth. He created you with dignity that disease can never take away. He loves you so much that He sent Jesus to give you complete freedom from shame. You are never covered with shame when you reflect the radiant beauty of Christ.

Pray: Dear God, thank You for creating me with dignity and worth. Take my feelings of discomfort and embarrassment about my disease, and use them to impart greater compassion for others who suffer. Fill me with the knowledge of who I am in Christ. Amen.

Embrace: Shame will never cover me when I reflect the radiant beauty of Jesus Christ; I possess dignity and worth that illness cannot take away.

Worship: "You Define Me" by Kim Walker-Smith

Claiming Every Benefit

—————————

Praise the LORD, my soul, and forget not all his benefits.
—*Psalm 103:2*

Those of us with medical-insurance providers make sure to claim all the benefits our policies allow; to do otherwise would be foolish. You may not have medical insurance, but you will always have a provider who gives you great benefits. God extends love and compassion when you feel alone. He provides direction and wisdom during all your medical decisions. Remember the benefits that you have in the Lord, and then claim them by thanking God for them.

Preventive health care helps us defend against developing further medical issues. God's Word teaches us how to fortify our thoughts as well. Safeguard your mind and spirit from hopelessness by rejoicing in the goodness of the Lord. Rejoicing will guard your soul and strengthen your faith to withstand every hardship. Which of God's benefits will you claim through praise today?[2]

Pray: Dear God, thank You that I have eternal benefits because You are my provider. You are loving, merciful, and good. You are compassionate and kind. Thank You for the benefit of salvation that is mine in Christ; it is the best insurance plan by far. I love You, Lord. Amen.

Embrace: My provider has benefits for me to claim today.

Worship: "10,000 Reasons (Bless the Lord) (Live)" by Matt Redman

Every Moment of Your Life

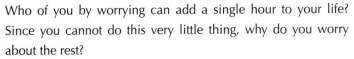

Who of you by worrying can add a single hour to your life? Since you cannot do this very little thing, why do you worry about the rest?

—Luke 12:25–26

Living with health issues often feels like a full-time job. We go to doctors' appointments, wait at pharmacies, attend physical therapy, schedule the next set of tests or infusions—and then we start again the following week. It can feel overwhelming unless we train our minds to stay in the moment. God gives you everything you need in order to endure, precisely when you need it. Time does not constrain the One who created time; He already holds all the seconds that make up your life. You do not need to worry about your future, because God's goodness already reaches into all your days. His loving mercy stands ready to greet you during every moment of your life.

Pray: Dear God, thank You for helping me endure through every moment. I do not have to fear the future, because You are already there. Your goodness walks before me; You provide everything I need at the right time. Help me make the most of every moment that You give me. In Jesus's name, amen.

Embrace: I will not fear my future, because God's goodness is waiting there for me.

Worship: "Psalm 23 (Surely Goodness, Surely Mercy)" by Shane & Shane

Complaining Is Draining

––––––––––––––––––––

Do everything without grumbling or arguing.
—*Philippians 2:14*

I have a friend who is going through many health difficulties. She pours out a cascade of complaints every time I talk with her. But I have often done the same thing to others. I spew the toxic torrent of negativity and ingratitude onto them when I complain. Complaining drains bitterness onto others; it also drains any hope of genuine connection with them. We often complain when we want compassion or understanding about our illness from those around us. But a heart that overflows with grumbling has no room to receive comfort.

One complaint department is always open; it is the only place to present all your complaints. Take every problem and every dissatisfaction to God in prayer. Release your troubles by telling them to the Lord, and then fill up on the comfort of His love for you. Let your heart overflow with praise and thanksgiving so that a complaining spirit has no room to return.

Pray: Dear God, forgive me when I complain to others. Sometimes I just want someone to understand the pain I endure; I need comfort and compassion. But I recognize that excessive complaints will only drive people away. You are the only one who is fully equipped to carry my heavy load. Give me a spirit of praise that overflows to those around me. In Jesus's name, amen.

Embrace: I will take my complaints to the Lord in prayer and fill my spirit with praise so that they have no room to return.

Worship: "Trust in You (Radio Edit)" by Anthony Brown and group therAPy

A Little Healing Means a Lot

LORD my God, I called to you for help, and you healed me.
—*Psalm 30:2*

A small scar on my jaw reminds me of when I had chicken pox during college. The three-inch scar across my neck reminds me of the multiple surgeries and complications that followed a biopsy for cancer. The scar that spans the entire length of my left hand reminds me of two surgeries that followed a golf-cart accident. What do all these scars have in common? They are signs of healing. I no longer have chicken pox, biopsy complications, or a broken hand. Some of my scars are faint, so you might never notice them. But they each tell a tale of God's mercy in mending former health issues. Do you long for healing? Look at your scars; they are evidence of God's merciful healing power in your life. Recall God's faithfulness to you by recounting all the ways you have already been healed.

Pray: Dear God, forgive me when I forget all the ways You have already mended me. You are faithful. Help me see my scars as evidence of past healing. I remember that the scars on Your hands and feet are evidence of my greatest healing. Thank You for the wounds that healed me from the bondage of sin. I will put my trust in You today. Amen.

Embrace: I build great faith when I thank God for all the little ways He has already healed me.

Worship: "Evidence" by Josh Baldwin

Comfort for Weary Warriors

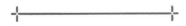

The horse is made ready for the day of battle, but victory rests
with the LORD.

—*Proverbs 21:31*

Fighting illness is exhausting, but weariness sets in when you believe that you alone are responsible for the success of your fight.
God created your life, and only He can sustain it. Are you weary from
battling illness? Then take comfort from His word to the weary and
worried Israelites as they faced a fight for their future:

> The LORD your God, who is going before you, will fight for you, as he
> did for you in Egypt, before your very eyes, and in the wilderness.
> There you saw how the LORD your God carried you, as a father carries
> his son, all the way you went until you reached this place. (Deuter-
> onomy 1:30–31)

The Lord will continue to help you fight your health battles. He
has carried you this far; you can trust Him to carry you through all
your days until He heals you completely by carrying you home.

Pray: Dear God, sometimes I am so entrenched in the war
against my illness that I forget I do not fight alone. Thank You
that You are by my side. Give me wisdom as I choose treatments
and make health decisions. You are in control of all my days, so
I can rest in Your arms and allow You to fight for me. In Jesus's
name, amen.

Embrace: I can rest from my health battles because the Lord fights for me.

Worship: "Battle Belongs" by Phil Wickham

Comparison Blocks Compassion

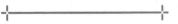

If you harbor bitter envy and selfish ambition in your hearts, do not boast about it or deny the truth.

—*James 3:14*

I was amazed by the outpouring of love during my difficult season of aggressive chemotherapy. I felt such support when I read encouraging comments on my Facebook page. But then I read the page of someone else who had cancer. She had hundreds of comments and photos of people wearing T-shirts to support her. Suddenly my twenty-three heartfelt, supportive comments melted into nothing. I felt envious when I should have been filled with compassion for someone else who was suffering.

Comparison takes your eyes off God's provision and purpose in your life. It creates envy that robs you of compassion and love for others. Have you compared yourself with others recently? Comparison may cause envy that destroys your peace, but confession and thanksgiving always restore it. Try them and see.

Pray: Dear God, forgive me when I compare myself or my circumstances with others. I recognize that You have a unique purpose for my life and have equipped me to fulfill it. Forgive me for wanting what You have allotted for others. Please restore my joy by helping me practice the discipline of thanksgiving. In Jesus's name, amen.

Embrace: When comparison steals contentment, confession and thanksgiving will always restore it.

Worship: "I Shall Not Want" by Audrey Assad

Catering to Illness

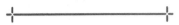

Behold, as the eyes of servants look to the hand of their master, and as the eyes of a maid to the hand of her mistress, so our eyes look to the LORD our God, until He is gracious and favorable toward us.

—*Psalm 123:2, AMP*

I love to watch Masterpiece television shows. The sets are opulent, particularly during dinner scenes in English manor houses. But the people next to the silver-laden table are often the most interesting to watch. The butler and waitstaff stand and watch for the mistress of the house to signal by lifting her hand so they can serve the next course. If they are distracted, are looking away, or have their eyes closed, they will miss the signal. Waiting on someone requires patience and humility. It also requires focus; we serve at the beck and call of whatever demands all our attention. I refuse to cater to the demands of illness. Instead, I will wait on God by placing my thoughts on Christ, my eyes on God's Word, and my hope in the gospel.

Pray: Dear God, help me not to be so distracted by my illness that I miss the movements of Your hand. You are preparing a feast for me, and You invite me to serve now and feast with You later. May I be still enough to hear You, wise enough to wait, and humble enough to obey. In Jesus's name, amen.

Embrace: I will pay full attention to the Lord by loving Him with all my mind, heart, soul, and strength.

Worship: "Love the Lord" by Lincoln Brewster

True Abundance

The thief comes only in order to steal and kill and destroy. I came that they may have and enjoy life, and have it in abundance [to the full, till it overflows].
—John 10:10, AMP

I bought into a dangerous lie when I first became sick. I mistakenly equated the abundant life of a believer with a physically active life. I had even been told as much by other well-meaning Christians. But abundant life is the spiritual life that begins when a believer accepts Jesus. Do you have Jesus? Then you have life in the Spirit that overflows within you, welling up to eternal life. A spiritual life in Christ is the only source of unending strength, peace, and joy in the midst of overwhelming health issues. Nothing can take away your true abundant life. It is an eternal gift that helps you endure illness. True abundance does not disappear or run out in the face of adversity. It equips you to live victoriously through it.

Pray: Dear God, thank You that Your gifts do not operate based on the state of my health. Continue to teach me truth that conquers all my despair. Thank You that I can have true abundant life because I have You. Help me pursue life in the Spirit so I will not be discouraged by the failings of my flesh. In Jesus's name, amen.

Embrace: Jesus gives me abundant life that starts now and lasts for eternity.

Worship: "Abundant Life" by Christ Our Life

Eternal Healing

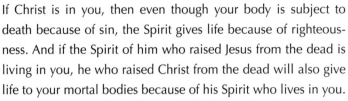

If Christ is in you, then even though your body is subject to death because of sin, the Spirit gives life because of righteousness. And if the Spirit of him who raised Jesus from the dead is living in you, he who raised Christ from the dead will also give life to your mortal bodies because of his Spirit who lives in you.
—Romans 8:10–11

When I read today's scripture, I am reminded that there is a reason for those moments when illness makes my body feel like it is dying. My earthly body will not live forever, so why am I surprised when it feels the sentence of mortality? My physical ailments are reminders that I need more than temporary healing—I need the eternal life that Jesus gives me. I will always pray for healing, but when I have Jesus, I have the sure hope of eternal healing: bodily restoration, transformation, and life forever in heaven. May every ache and pain, every weakness, and every health issue continually point me to my need for Jesus.

Pray: Dear God, please use my physical ailments to make me hunger for more than temporary healing. Let them continually point me to the hope of eternal healing. Thank You for sending Jesus to forgive my sins so that I can have eternal life in heaven. In Jesus's name, amen.

Embrace: My physical ailments are reminders that I need more than temporary healing—I need the hope of salvation that Jesus gives me.

Worship: "Light and Momentary" by For All Seasons

This Wasn't Part of My Plan

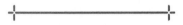

> We know [with great confidence] that God [who is deeply concerned about us] causes all things to work together [as a plan] for good for those who love God, to those who are called according to His plan and purpose.
> —*Romans 8:28, AMP*

When I was a little girl, I had a rotating list of careers that I wanted to pursue. Artist. Ballerina. Poet. Never once, when someone asked, did I answer that I wanted to grow up to be disabled by illness. Having chronic disease and cancer was never part of my plan.

Illness was likely never part of *your* plan either. Your health issues may have been a surprise to you, but they were not a surprise to God. He has already enacted a plan to bring good through them, amid them, and despite them. You can trust your loving creator to create blessing even out of brokenness. The same God whose resurrection power triumphed over death is implementing a powerfully good plan and purpose for your life.

Pray: Lord, You promise that You will work everything together for good for those who love You. I love You; help me trust You. Strengthen my faith by deepening my relationship with You. Thank You that I can trust Your plan for my life. My illness, pain, and suffering are not a surprise to You. You will help me through them and use them for my good. Amen.

Embrace: God has a plan to make all these things—illness, pain, and suffering—work for my good.

Worship: "Canvas and Clay (Live)" by Pat Barrett, featuring Ben Smith

Strength That Endures

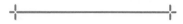

As they pass through the Valley of Baka, they make it a place of springs; the autumn rains also cover it with pools. They go from strength to strength, till each appears before God in Zion.

—Psalm 84:6–7

Do you ever feel as though you are fighting one illness after another? Living with a chronic disease does not exempt you from receiving another diagnosis. It does not even exempt you from catching a cold. It is difficult to endure when one health issue follows another. Declining health can lead to increasing despair. You may experience grief, pain, and tears. But God will fill your valley of tears with pools of blessing. He will guide you through each difficulty and give you moments of respite along the way. Every health issue that you encounter becomes another opportunity to receive the strength that endures.

Pray: Dear God, thank You for giving me the strength to endure illness. Help me see the ways You have filled my valley of tears with pools of blessing. They will always reflect Your goodness and Your love for me. I can travel through anything I face, because You give me strength for the journey. Amen.

Embrace: All my strength is bound up in Christ; He gives it to me when I need it.

Worship: "You Hold It All Together" by All Sons & Daughters, featuring Leslie Jordan and David Leonard

Truly Knowing God

Those who know your name trust in you, for you, LORD, have never forsaken those who seek you.
—Psalm 9:10

Faith in God's character—truly knowing Him—is the secret to remaining steadfast during my health issues. Illness cannot dim my hope when I am convinced of His goodness, supremacy, and watchful care over my life. He sifts all my circumstances through His loving hands, so I can stop struggling against them and start living victoriously despite them. I am not looking back—or even ahead—but instead facing each day with the grace that God has apportioned. Living by faith is the only way to withstand living with illness.

Pray: Dear God, thank You for the gift of faith. Sometimes, like the father in the gospel of Mark, I must cry, "Lord, I believe; help my unbelief!" (9:24, NKJV). Help me grow in my relationship with Jesus. Teach me that my circumstances and health challenges are not barometers of Your love for me. Help me know You so that I will trust You. Amen.

Embrace: To know God is to trust Him.

Worship: "Abide (Live)" by the Worship Initiative, featuring Aaron Williams and Dwell Songs

Growing Pains

I am sure that God who began the good work within you will keep right on helping you grow in his grace until his task within you is finally finished on that day when Jesus Christ returns.

—Philippians 1:6, TLB

Three of my family members had severe life-altering health issues while I was undergoing treatment for cancer. I temporarily suspended treatments so I could have the strength to support my loved ones, and God held me together even as I fell apart during the heartbreaking devastation of this season. He used the health challenges that broke all our hearts to create new spaces within them. Our empty spaces ached for healing of body, mind, and spirit. But these spaces also held room for the promise of future restoration and deliverance.

It turns out that our hearts were too small to receive all that Jesus had to give us; they had to be broken to make space for more faith, more love, and more compassion. We learned that the Lord never allows destruction only to leave us in devastation. So if you feel broken apart and destroyed, then just wait—God is doing a mighty work in you. Growing pains are evidence that you are enlarging your capacity to receive the abundance of Christ.

Pray: Lord, take my broken and empty spaces. Help me hold Your promise of future restoration within them. Fill me with Your abundance. Create a new heart and a new spirit within me. Amen.

Embrace: Growing pains are evidence that I am enlarging my capacity to receive the abundance of Christ.

Worship: "Gracefully Broken" by Tasha Cobbs Leonard

Fragrant Offerings

I call to you, LORD, come quickly to me; hear me when I call to you. May my prayer be set before you like incense; may the lifting up of my hands be like the evening sacrifice.
—*Psalm 141:1–2*

Today when I bowed my head to pray, I began to smell the lovely floral and apricot hand cream I was wearing. It made me feel happy. It was a delicate whiff of beauty floating up to my nostrils. I am reminded that our prayers are the same for God. They are like incense, rising to the throne of God and filling His presence with their sweetness. Our cries, praises, and petitions are fragrant offerings for the Lord.

Pray: Lord, thank You that my prayers are precious to You. Help me pray continually and give thanks to You throughout my day. Remind me that my words do not have to be perfect; You intercede when I do not know what to say. Help me never to take it for granted that the God of the universe wants to communicate with me. In Your name, amen.

Embrace: My prayers are a beautiful and powerful act of worship.

Worship: "Here I Am to Worship" by William McDowell

Where Are You Going?

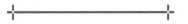

Where can I go from your Spirit? Where can I flee from your presence? If I go up to the heavens, you are there; if I make my bed in the depths, you are there. If I rise on the wings of the dawn, if I settle on the far side of the sea, even there your hand will guide me, your right hand will hold me fast.

—Psalm 139:7–10

Where are you going this week? I am going to my oncologist's office. Next week I will visit my physical therapist. The current regulations at both medical clinics state that visitors are not allowed. But I never go alone, for the Lord travels with me. His presence calms my anxiety as I drive closer to the oncology clinic. His peace envelops me in the waiting room. His compassion flows through me as I pray for the patients around me. He is always with me.

The Lord is with you wherever you go today. He will be with you during all the days ahead. He will never leave you. You are not going alone to medical appointments, surgeries, or treatments. The Lord will meet you wherever you go, and He will usher you through anything you face. He will never forsake you.

Pray: Dear God, thank You that I do not have to be alone during the difficulties of illness. Give me Your comfort when medical issues make me anxious. Envelop me with Your peace when I am afraid. Fill me with Your loving compassion for everyone I meet along the way. In Jesus's name, amen.

Embrace: Illness is the specific address where God is going to meet me.

Worship: "I Am Not Alone (Live)" by Kari Jobe

Temporary Residence

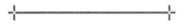

All these people were still living by faith when they died. They did not receive the things promised; they only saw them and welcomed them from a distance, admitting that they were foreigners and strangers on earth.

—*Hebrews 11:13*

Being faced with sudden illness is like waking up in a country that you never wanted to visit. Those of us with chronic illness know that our visit to the land of medical issues has become an involuntary extended stay. We are always seeking ways to rejoin the healthy world, but the fact is that we already belong to a better world. Residence in the land of illness will always be temporary. Health issues reinforce the beautiful truth that we are made for more than this world. We can patiently endure pain, health issues, and any other difficulty because faith gives us the perspective to see eternal hope.[3]

Pray: Dear God, thank You for the examples of faithful people in the Bible. They show us how to patiently endure hardship. I can look ahead with hope, no matter what comes, because You have already secured my future for eternity. Thank You for sending Jesus to die for me so my pain will not last forever. Thank You for all the healing that is mine in Christ. Amen.

Embrace: I can patiently endure illness because it is temporary; faith gives me the perspective to see eternal hope.

Worship: "I Can Only Imagine" by MercyMe

The Greatest Exchange

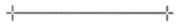

What good will it be for someone to gain the whole world, yet forfeit their soul? Or what can anyone give in exchange for their soul?

—*Matthew 16:26*

A spiritual life in Christ is a series of exchanges. We trade the bondage of sin and shame for the freedom of forgiveness. We exchange the death that our sins deserve for the gift of eternal life that Jesus freely gives us. This is possible only because Jesus made the greatest exchange of all: He sacrificed His life to gain eternal life for us when He died on the cross. He paid the price to redeem us so that we could make one final miraculous exchange. Those of us who have given our lives to Jesus will trade a broken body for a fully healed body when we die. Have you entrusted your life to Jesus Christ? Release your doubts by receiving Him through faith. It is, by far, the most significant exchange you will ever make.

Pray: Lord, thank You for exchanging Your life for my soul. I do not need to work for salvation, because You already did the work. Today, help me embrace the truth that my sins are fully forgiven through Jesus's sacrifice. Thank You that I will one day exchange this broken body for one that will be fully healed for eternity. Amen.

Embrace: I will exchange my doubts for faith because Jesus exchanged His life for mine.

Worship: "Divine Exchange" by Charity Gayle, featuring Corey Voss

Prayers Are Always Welcome

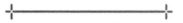

Let us then approach God's throne of grace with confidence, so that we may receive mercy and find grace to help us in our time of need.

—*Hebrews 4:16*

In the midst of a frightening diagnosis or ongoing pain, it is easy to believe the lie that God does not hear our cries for help. But not having our prayers answered the way we want or in our preferred time frame only means that we are not God! It does not mean that He does not love us or hear us. He sent Jesus to die so you could have eternal life with Him. Why would God want to live with you for eternity but refuse to hear you right now? He wants you to communicate with Him through prayer. Pray even when you do not feel like it, because that is when you need to pray the most. Just tell God what is on your heart. There is no right way to pray, but the Lord's Prayer (below) is a great place to begin.

Pray: Jesus taught His disciples to pray by saying, "Our Father in heaven, may your name be kept holy. May your Kingdom come soon. May your will be done on earth, as it is in heaven. Give us today the food we need, and forgive us our sins, as we have forgiven those who sin against us. And don't let us yield to temptation, but rescue us from the evil one" (Matthew 6:9–13, NLT).

Embrace: God always welcomes and hears my prayers.

Worship: "What a Friend We Have in Jesus" by The Worship Initiative and Shane & Shane, featuring Hannah Hardin

Are You Exhausted?

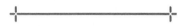

I will refresh the weary and satisfy the faint.
—*Jeremiah 31:25*

Aggressive lymphoma made me the most fatigued I have ever been in my life. I already knew that living with illness was exhausting, but I learned that fighting illness *so you can live* is exhausting in an entirely different way. The cure for both kinds of exhaustion extends beyond the realm of physical rest. Spiritual restoration is the key to enduring the bone-level fatigue of illness.

What do you do to rest after a day filled with treatments or medical appointments? Watching the news or getting lost in social media will only heap the weight of the world on you. Do you feel genuinely rested when you pursue these activities? Not only will they never bring you the rest that you crave, but these idle pursuits will further deplete you. Give your spirit a rest from the world by filling up with the things that satisfy you. Before you sleep, rejuvenate yourself through prayer, praise music, and sermons that bathe you in truth. These spiritual pursuits strengthen your spirit to endure the exhaustion of illness.

Pray: Dear God, help me pursue Your rest when I am weary. Give me the wisdom and self-control to guard my spirit against being burdened by the weight of the world. Help me restore my soul by pursuing the things that satisfy. I will rest in You, and I will endure because You are my strength. In Jesus's name, amen.

Embrace: Idle pursuits will exhaust me, but godly pursuits will restore me.

Worship: "Press On" by Selah

A Marvelous Meal

This section offers the hearty satisfaction of spiritual sustenance. Longer than the entries in "A Satisfying Snack" but shorter than those in "A Fabulous Feast," these medium-length entries are just right for days when you have the energy and ability to focus on reading a slightly longer devotion.

By his divine power, God has given us everything we need for living a godly life. We have received all of this by *coming to know him,* the one who CALLED US to himself by means of his marvelous glory and excellence.

—2 Peter 1:3, NLT

Desperate for Answers

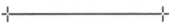

Trust in and rely confidently on the LORD with all your heart and do not rely on your own insight or understanding.
—*Proverbs 3:5*, AMP

I was frightened when I began having health issues. A slew of symptoms led to visits with multiple doctors. I visited a gastroenterologist for stomach issues, and I consulted with a neurologist and a rheumatologist because of my widespread pain. Gynecologists performed surgery after surgery. My urologist, not one to be left out, also performed procedures. My body seemed to be breaking down a piece at a time, and each piece had a doctor assigned to it.

My father is a physician. He pored over medical journals to find a cure for my health issues. A steady stream of research studies filled my inbox as he shared his findings. I eagerly consumed this knowledge because I was desperate to find a way to heal my broken body. But the all-consuming quest to heal my body began to break my spirit. What started as a journey to find answers brought me an answer I never expected. I learned that an unhealthy fixation on my broken pieces will never result in healing; it will only break me further.

After decades of ever-increasing illness, I now recognize that the Great Physician is in charge of my mind, body, spirit, and soul. He is able to heal every part of me. I have peace when I spend more time praying to my healer than searching the internet for healing. I can rest in my search for answers when I trust the God who knows every answer.

Pray: Dear God, You are the one who knows the reasons for my health issues, and You know the solutions. Help me trust You as I search for answers. Guide me on Your path. Give me patient trust as I wait for healing. In Jesus's name, amen.

Embrace: An unhealthy fixation on my brokenness will never result in healing; it will only break me further.

Practice: Turn to Psalm 121, and read it aloud to remember that you can trust God with your life. Commit it to memory, or write it on a card to keep nearby.

Worship: "Just Be Held" by Casting Crowns

Pressed Juice

A good man brings good things out of the good stored up in him,
and an evil man brings evil things out of the evil stored up in
him.

—*Matthew 12:35*

I must let the trials that God allows in my life bring forth sweetness
in my character. When pressed, sour grapes will yield sour juice,
and sweet ones will produce sweet juice. Likewise, when hardship
presses me, the thoughts I have nurtured will determine what flows
out of me.

It was so easy to be kind when I was not in chronic pain. My children knew their mother's ready smile. I laughed often, and my giggle
was well known to my friends. I was pressed by stress on occasion, as
everyone is, but it was not the industrial-strength press intended to
bring every last drop of juice out of the grape. Pain is both that
industrial-strength press and the heat that spoils and sours the
grape. It is difficult to bring forth sweetness under the pressure of
pain. But with God, all things are possible, even the seemingly im-
possible task of bringing succulent sweetness out of agonizing affliction.

So I surrender my frustrations to the Lord. I allow Him to crucify
my bitterness about my illness when I die to my supposed *right* to be
bitter. Negative and ruminating thoughts die a quick death in the
light of Jesus's love for me. His love conquers all, even self-pitying
thoughts about my pain and illness. I spend time with Jesus, and I
ask His forgiveness for not trusting Him to help me through each
pain-filled day. Repentance empties my heart of the bitterness that
sours, so I am finally ready to soak up the warmth of His mercy and

the comfort of His love. Spending time with Jesus restores sweet contentment to my soul.

Pray: Lord, You know the discouraging and fearful thoughts I often have about my pain and illness. Grant me the wisdom to recognize that doubt and discontent create fertile ground for despair. Give me the tools to cultivate life-giving thoughts and attitudes. May they grow into words of healing for those around me. Open my eyes to see that illness may act as the press but Your hand does the pressing. In Jesus's name, amen.

Embrace: Spending time with Jesus restores sweet contentment to my soul.

Ponder: Have you experienced any bitterness over your health struggles? Confess it to God. Spend time in prayer, and ask Him to restore your soul.

Worship: "I Surrender All" by Joey + Rory

Moving Forward During a Setback

One thing I do: Forgetting what is behind and straining toward what is ahead, I press on toward the goal to win the prize for which God has called me heavenward in Christ Jesus.
—*Philippians 3:13–14*

Those of us with a complicated health history know that a new illness triggers old memories. The pain, fatigue, and misery of a health setback are bodily reminders of all the other times we have suffered from illness. New health issues are emissaries from the land of illness; they capture us and attempt to drag us back to that place we so desperately hoped to leave. A setback ushers us back into the world that we tried, by all means possible, to escape.

It is true that becoming sick is difficult for everyone. But it is grueling for those who have lived long years fighting battle after battle against sickness. It is discouraging when all your health gains seem to disappear in a heartbeat. Making every effort to be healthy does not always ensure good health, so placing all your hopes in the state of your health is no hope at all. Setbacks can make us feel like giving up, because it is never enough to pursue health. We must pursue life.

God gives us everything we need for life—for true life—no matter the state of our health. His divine power enables us to live with hope, strength, and perseverance in every circumstance. When you have Jesus, you have all you need to navigate the difficulties of illness. He is with you always, eagerly pursuing you with goodness and merciful kindness. You can move forward during a health setback because you have sure hope that is not bound by circumstance, strength that is stronger than you feel, and patient endurance to bear absolutely anything that comes your way.

Pray: Dear Lord, I am discouraged by my illness today. I am weary. You promise that those who hope in You will renew their strength. I need that strength today, Lord, so I place all my hope in You. Use this time in my life to refine me; help me rely on faith instead of feelings. Thank You that setbacks are opportunities to grow in faith by relying more fully on Your grace. Lord, I praise You that nothing, not even poor health, can separate me from Your love. In Jesus's name, amen.

Embrace: My health setbacks are opportunities for my faith to grow.

Ponder: It is common to feel despair or hopelessness after experiencing a health setback. Have you ever been blindsided by additional health issues? How did you cope with your disappointment or discouragement?

Worship: "Shoulders" by For King and Country

Special Care Packages

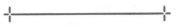

My God will meet all your needs according to the riches of his glory in Christ Jesus.

—Philippians 4:19

Our three children loved going to summer camp for a few weeks each year. The camp always provided a list of items that each camper would need for the adventures ahead. They even instructed us to send letters and special care packages so that our children would be comforted if they were homesick. We made many trips to the store to buy the items on the packing list. As loving parents, we carefully made sure they were well equipped for camp. From bug spray to sunscreen to shower shoes, we packed up everything they would need. Sometimes their suitcases were so full that they later had to search diligently to discover what we had packed for them.

Do you ever worry that you will not have what you need to endure living with illness? Your health issues may be a surprise to you, but they are not a surprise to God. Like any loving parent, your Father has provided everything necessary for the journey ahead. Unpack the promises in your Bible to discover what He has given you. When you are homesick for the life you used to lead, ask Him to bring special care packages that provide comfort. The encouragement of a friend, the wisdom of a timely Scripture verse, and the beauty of a sunset are all perfectly packaged to give you whatever you need at that moment. God has planned good things for you both today and in your future. Even your most challenging days with illness cannot keep His mercies from finding you.

Pray: Dear God, there are days when the hardship of illness weighs heavily on me. I cannot do this alone; I need You to equip me thoroughly. Lead me to discover the truth that speaks to my situation. You have packed so much for me in Scripture. Help me unpack all the promises You have for me; do not let me miss anything. Thank You that You have not left me alone but have given me the Holy Spirit as my comforter to instruct me and strengthen me. Thank You for all the ways You provide for me. In Jesus's name, amen.

Embrace: I will discover what God has provided for me when I unpack the promises in Scripture.

Ponder: Would a loving parent refuse to equip a child for camp when they had the means to do so? Why or why not? Would your heavenly Father allow you to travel through health issues without giving you what you need? Thank God for packing up so many promises and blessings for you to discover.

Worship: "Good Good Father" by Chris Tomlin

The Destination Will Be Worth It

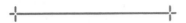

You have persevered and have endured hardships for my name,
and have not grown weary. . . . To the one who is victorious, I
will give the right to eat from the tree of life, which is in the
paradise of God.

—*Revelation 2:3, 7*

Traveling is difficult when you have chronic pain or illness. Packing a suitcase can exacerbate pain, and extensive preparations for travel cause complete exhaustion before you even leave your house. For those with health issues, moving through an airport and spending long hours on a plane can make going on a dream vacation feel like a nightmare. I learned that firsthand when my husband and I traveled to Hawaii last year. In all my daydreams about visiting Hawaii, I had never actually considered the physical toll it would take to get there. It seemed the painful hours spent in multiple airports and airplanes would never end. But they did end, and after a day of rest, I found myself swimming in crystal-clear water and feeling like a child again as its buoyancy relieved my pain. It turned out that the temporary troubles of traveling to paradise were worth it.

Paradise is the final destination for all who have received Jesus Christ as Lord. But hardships can block our eternal perspective, causing us to lose sight of true hope. What if I had decided that Hawaii could not possibly exist because the journey to get there was too difficult? That is what we do when we allow suffering to destroy faith in God's promises. What if I had looked around the dimly lit airplane and begun to believe I would never leave its stuffy cabin? Imagine my discouragement! But that is what we do when we believe that trials and hardships will never end.

Has suffering caused you to lose sight of the future God has planned for you? An eternal perspective gives us the hope we need to continue the journey. You do not travel alone; the Holy Spirit is your advocate, counselor, and helper in this life and your guarantee of eternal life. God has uniquely equipped you with everything you need to persevere. Remember, you have a way through anything you face when you have Jesus. Keep going. The destination He is preparing for you will be worth it.

Pray: Dear God, forgive me when I become so overwhelmed by the difficulties of the journey that I forget to rejoice and look forward to the destination. I can trust Your plan for my life, no matter the hardship, because You have promised never to leave me or forsake me. I will persevere because I bear Your name. I will endure because You have given me everything I need for this life. I can do all things because You strengthen me. Thank You for helping me. In Jesus's name, amen.

Embrace: I can keep going because the destination Jesus is preparing for me will be worth it.

Ponder: Have you ever told yourself that your illness or pain will last forever? How do thoughts like that affect your outlook or ability to endure? What can you do to regain a better perspective?

Worship: "Worth It All" by the Brooklyn Tabernacle Choir

Marching Through the Battlefield

O my soul, march on with strength.
—*Judges 5:21, AMP*

Have you ever noticed that people use terms of warfare to describe illness? We say that someone is *fighting* the flu or that they are *battling* depression. We describe cancer as having *invaded* us, and when we are successful in treating it, we say that we have *won the fight*. Managing chronic illness often feels like living through battle after battle. Facing sudden severe health issues can feel like an all-out war. What do you need after such a fight? In the Old Testament, after Deborah was an eyewitness to a victorious but horrific battle, she declared, "O my soul, march on with strength" (Judges 5:21, AMP). It is not enough to win a battle; you must have the strength left to march off the battlefield.

The fight against cancer is exhausting. It took aggressive chemotherapy, repeated surgeries, and numerous hospitalizations before I achieved remission. My battle against cancer seemed to be over, but I had to continue the attack to ensure it would not return. I desperately wanted to declare victory and leave the battlefield, but a longer-lasting truce with cancer meant I needed years of additional treatment. Even though I won the battle, I needed strength to march through the rest of the battlefield.

Where are you in your fight with illness? Are you still deep in combat, or are you celebrating a series of victories? Take your eyes off the battlefield, as Deborah did, and remind your soul to march on with the strength God gives you. Have you heard the saying that preparation is half the battle? Prepare yourself for victory by strengthening your soul with truth from God's Word. Determine not to give up. One day you will be able to share your testimony of God's provision and power with those who are fighting their own battles. Keep marching, my friend.

Pray: Dear God, I am weary from battling illness, but I know that You give strength to the weary. I ask for that mighty power today. Fill me with Your Holy Spirit. You are my helper and the one who fights for me. Thank You that I do not face any battle alone. I can march onward through these trials because You are my strength. In Jesus's name, amen.

Embrace: I will prepare myself for victory by strengthening my soul and marching on through the battlefield.

Practice: Write a testimony of God's faithfulness during your battle with health issues. Add to it daily. Look for opportunities to share your testimony with others facing similar struggles.

Worship: "The Battle Is the Lord's" by Yolanda Adams

Suffering Is Never in Vain

————————————

Though he brings grief, he will show compassion, so great is his unfailing love. For he does not willingly bring affliction or grief to anyone.

—Lamentations 3:32–33

Streams in the Desert by L. B. Cowman is one of my favorite devotionals. The inspiring passages often challenge me to rethink the purpose of suffering:

George Matheson, the well-known blind preacher of Scotland, once said, "My dear God, I have never thanked You for my thorns. I have thanked [Y]ou a thousand times for my roses but not once for my thorns. I have always looked forward to the place where I will be rewarded for my cross, but I have never thought of my cross as a present glory itself.

"Teach me, O Lord, to glory in my cross. Teach me the value of my thorns. Show me how I have climbed to You through the path of pain."[1]

Have you ever wondered why Jesus had to wear a crown of thorns? It was not random cruelty; it held great significance. The consequences of Adam's sin included a curse on all creation: "Cursed is the ground because of you; in pain you shall eat of it all the days of your life; *thorns* and thistles it shall bring forth for you" (Genesis 3:17–18, ESV, emphasis added). The crown of thorns symbolized the fact that Jesus, our king, took the entire curse on Himself. None of His suffering was in vain; it perfectly fulfilled prophecy and paid the debt for all the sins of humanity. His great suffering was part of a greater plan.

The God who suffered greatly for you does not look lightly on your suffering. You can cry out to Him amid your pain because He has great compassion for you. You are precious to the Lord. None of your suffering is in vain. It is propelling you toward an eternal glory that far outweighs every trouble and trial. You may not understand the reasons for your pain and hardship, but you can trust the Author of life with this scene of your story.

Pray: Dear God, thank You for suffering the pain of the cross so I do not have to experience eternal suffering. I may not understand the purpose for my pain, but I trust that You will use it for good. Help me trust You with the outcome even if I do not understand the process. Sometimes it feels as though my pain will never end, but You have promised eternal restoration and healing. Give me eternal perspective and patient perseverance to live out this portion of my story. Encourage and strengthen me, Lord, so I can endure no matter what comes my way. In Jesus's name, amen.

Embrace: I trust the Author of life to weave redemption into every part of my story.

Ponder: Jesus did not suffer anything in vain; every part of His crucifixion had a redemptive purpose. In what ways do you think God will use your suffering to bring about greater redemption in your life? How does trusting Him with the entire story help you endure this chapter of your life?

Worship: "God's Not Done with You" by Tauren Wells

The Invisible Highway

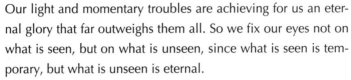

Our light and momentary troubles are achieving for us an eternal glory that far outweighs them all. So we fix our eyes not on what is seen, but on what is unseen, since what is seen is temporary, but what is unseen is eternal.
— *2 Corinthians 4:17–18*

Over the past few years, my husband and I have made numerous trips to MD Anderson Cancer Center for my oncology appointments. We never seem to leave our home in Austin on time, so we often arrive in Houston during rush hour. Have you ever driven in Houston during rush-hour traffic? The highway is bumper-to-bumper, with the cars stretching on for miles in both directions. One day, tired of travel and eager to get to the hotel to rest, I remarked that I wished we had an invisible highway so we could drive above all the cars and go directly to our hotel. Then I was struck by the realization that faith does this for us. Faith shows us the invisible so we can rise above the visible, and its final destination is a glorious place of rest.

Have your health issues ever seemed like a traffic jam, with one symptom after another keeping you from easily traveling through life? Chronic pain can shift your focus until all you think about is the sensation of pain. After all, we experience this world through our physical senses. But we must develop the spiritual sense of faith if we are to see beyond our temporary trials. Unshakable faith is produced when we read God's Word, believe it, and obey it. We see unseen realities more clearly when we fix our eyes on Jesus. Health issues tempt us to focus on the temporal; fixing our eyes on Jesus gives us an eternal perspective that puts illness in its proper place.

Pray: Dear Lord, strengthen my faith so it is stronger than my feelings. Teach me how to fix my thoughts on You when I am overwhelmed by pain or illness. Please help me learn and obey Your Word so it will saturate every part of my life. I need You. Open the eyes of my heart so I will know the true hope I have in Jesus Christ. Thank You that I do not have to endure this life alone; thank You for Your comfort and strength. In Jesus's name, amen.

Embrace: Faith shows me the invisible so I can rise above the visible, and its final destination is a glorious place of rest.

Ponder: "Health issues tempt us to focus on the temporal; fixing our eyes on Jesus gives us an eternal perspective that puts illness in its proper place." How have you found this to be true in your life?

Worship: "Turn Your Eyes upon Jesus" by Lauren Daigle

My Healer Knows Best

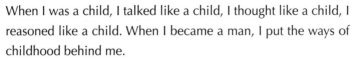

When I was a child, I talked like a child, I thought like a child, I reasoned like a child. When I became a man, I put the ways of childhood behind me.
—*1 Corinthians 13:11*

I order everything available on the medical menu when I am voraciously hungry for healing. I have taken medications, flown out of state to see doctors, attended physical therapy, been anointed with oil and prayed over, received acupuncture, participated in biofeedback, gone to chiropractors, been placed on special diets, received chemo and biologics, had transfusions, endured unbelievable surgeries, had my arm hooked up to IV infusions, had countless nerve blocks, bought supplements, and the list goes on and on because the menu is both exhaustive and exhausting. God is my healer, but I assumed it was my job to find the right vehicle through which He would perform my healing. The belief that physical healing must be His best for me has kept me on a never-ending search for it.

Today I had a new thought: *What if God's best for me is far more than I've ever imagined? What if it involves something different from my being healed and going back to an active lifestyle? What if God has greater plans for me than better health?* Perhaps He has given me supreme weakness so His power will be evident in my life. God's love for me will not allow pain and illness to break me simply to leave me in my shattered state. He always gives abundance; He will surely give me a life of purpose and hope despite any disease that tries to destroy me. In her book *Lessons I Learned in the Dark,* Jennifer Rothschild told a story in which her young son said of her blindness, "If God healed you here on earth, you might love earth more, and heaven is best."[2] How very wise. Our healer knows what is best for each of us, even as gut-wrenchingly difficult as it may be to accept. We must lean into Him and trust His ways, even when we cannot fathom His purpose.

Pray: Dear God, my search for healing has been exhausting. It is so difficult to know what steps to take to find the answers to my condition. Please guide me and give me the patience to trust Your timing. You are my maker, so You have a plan for me. You are my healer, so I continue to pray for healing. Help me trust You in everything You have allowed. Your plan for my life is best, even when it involves difficulty or suffering. Give me knowledge, understanding, and mature faith that endures. I love You. Amen.

Embrace: God always gives abundance; He will surely give me a life of purpose and hope despite any disease.

Ponder: Have you ever been told that it is God's will for every believer to be physically healed during this lifetime? If so, how has this shaped your beliefs about God or healing?

Worship: "Trust in You" by Lauren Daigle

A Tool of Transformation

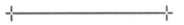

We all, who with unveiled faces contemplate the Lord's glory,
are being transformed into his image with ever-increasing glory,
which comes from the Lord, who is the Spirit.
—*2 Corinthians 3:18*

God graciously provides healthy ways to cope when pain over-
whelms me and makes me long to escape my hurting body. I
can reach out and ask someone to pray for me. I can meditate on
Scripture, listen to an encouraging audiobook, or play gospel music.
I can take an Epsom salt bath or perform a breathing exercise that
helps my pain.

But sometimes I choose to cope with pain by focusing on a mindless television show that I never would have watched before illness
struck. The truth is that mindless television is never mindless; it will
always influence my thoughts. Others who are afflicted with pain
may choose to overmedicate or sleep excessively in their attempts to
break free of it. The escape methods may vary, but choosing anything
that dishonors God will always lead to greater suffering.

When pain and suffering flood our lives, we become drowning
people with decisions to make. Will you reach out to the nearest device to help you float above water—even if you know it will ultimately
drag you under? Or will you rely on the Lord and resist the temptation to get into a sinking lifeboat? The things we depend on while
drowning in suffering reveal which "gods" we still turn to when we
turn away from God. Pain and suffering expose the truth about our
faith, allowing us to develop faith that is true.

What have pain and suffering revealed in your life? Are you
tempted to use your illness to excuse poor choices or sinful behavior?

Have you sometimes noticed a temptation toward self-pity or comparison? The apostle Peter warns us, "Be alert and of sober mind. Your enemy the devil prowls around like a roaring lion looking for someone to devour" (1 Peter 5:8). There is no true comfort in cuddling up with a roaring lion. Don't give the enemy a foothold in your battle with health issues. Let's refuse to be devoured by his tactics and strive instead for life-giving transformation.

Your heart is already "uncovered and laid bare before the eyes of him to whom we must give account" (Hebrews 4:13). So confess any poor habits, wrong choices, and negative character traits that your suffering may have revealed. Let your health issues be some of the tools God uses to refine your character and transform you into the image of Christ.

Pray: Dear God, sometimes I do not recognize the person I have become since illness struck. I confess that there are times I have been impatient, short-tempered, or quick to grasp anything that makes me feel better. Please forgive me for when I have turned away from You. Expose any sin that is keeping me from being filled with Your Spirit. Restore me and guide me; help me take the path that leads to life. Thank You for the forgiveness that is mine in Jesus Christ. Thank You for using even the difficult things in my life for good as You transform me into a new creation in Christ. In Jesus's name, amen.

Embrace: Suffering exposes the truth about my faith so I can develop faith that is true.

Ponder: What are you likely to turn to for relief from pain or illness? Has that helped enrich your life, or has it caused more issues for you? If you have turned to harmful thoughts, behaviors, or substances, please seek help from your physician. See the Resources section in the back of the book for additional help. You are worth it.

Worship: "Known" by Tauren Wells

Turn to the Table

✛━━━━━━━━━━━━━━✛

You prepare a table before me in the presence of my enemies.
—*Psalm 23:5*

The fight against pain, disease, and possibly even death can lead to an all-out war against illness. We fight with all we have in us. But there is a secret to winning this war: Do not allow the enemy of your soul to dictate your battle plan, and do not listen to him. He speaks the language of hopelessness so you will feel defeated. He whispers, "Your life will be one painful procedure after another. You will never escape crippling fatigue and disability. Cancer will spread; the pain will spread."

But there is a spread that no enemy can touch. Jesus offers a table of abundant provision with everything you need for victory. Do not allow your enemies to distract you from it. Turn to the table and feast. Then loudly declare, "I was parched; Jesus filled me with living water that refreshes my weary soul. I was famished; Jesus gave me Himself. He is the Bread of Life that strengthens and sustains me. He invites me to abide with Him, and He restores me until my cup of blessing runs over." The enemies of your body and soul may still be ready for battle, but you are strengthened for victory when you turn to the table. Jesus gives you everything you need in order to win.

Pray: Dear God, thank You for Your abundant provision for me. It amazes me that You loved me enough to send Jesus to die in my place so I could have the final victory of eternal life with You in heaven. Thank You for continuing to provide everything

I need in order to endure. You give me all I need for spiritual victory. Open the eyes of my heart so I may know the hope to which You have called me. Fill me with Your Holy Spirit to sustain me and guide me. Help me grow in my relationship with Jesus Christ so I can endure pain and illness. I love You, Lord. Amen.

Embrace: I will not allow the enemy to distract me from Jesus's abundant provision.

Ponder: Read 1 Corinthians 11:23–26. We turn to the Lord's Table when we take communion. Have your health issues prevented you from regularly receiving communion? If so, how can you remedy this?

Worship: "Abundantly More" by North Point Worship, featuring Seth Condrey

Accommodate Hope

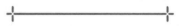

It is God who works in you to will and to act in order to fulfill his
good purpose.

—*Philippians 2:13*

Have you ever eaten store-bought meals or cereal for dinner because pain or fatigue prevented you from cooking? Are there certain chores that you have stopped doing altogether? Everything from the meals we eat to the chores we accomplish can be dictated by pain, fatigue, brain fog, and disability. Life becomes reduced to the basics when simple tasks require enormous determination. Our lives are changed, little by little, as we make accommodations to adjust to life with chronic illness.

Eventually, we begin to accept the limitations of illness as our new normal. There is freedom in acceptance, but there is a fine line between the acceptance that embraces a new reality and the resignation that gives in to it. Acceptance opens the door to perseverance in finding ways to live well despite illness; resignation closes all doors in an attempt to safeguard against any further illness, pain, or fatigue. Acceptance must lead us away from the roadblock of resignation and into the pathway of perseverance if we are to thrive amid health challenges.

If you have lived any amount of time with chronic illness, you have likely given in to a defeated mindset without even realizing it. Have you ever stayed in bed because you feared that activity would make your pain worse? Have you stopped having visitors over in an attempt to prevent fatigue? Surrendering to the fear of greater illness will lead to hopelessness. Surrender instead to the God who gives you hope. Remember that He can bring new opportunities to areas of your life that seem closed off by illness. Your story is not over; the God who began a good work in you is in the middle of completing it. Life may change to accommodate illness, but the God who never changes is still at work in your life.

Pray: Dear God, forgive me when I make room in my life for the work of illness but neglect to leave space for You to work. Show me the wonder of Your great love as You strengthen my hope and increase my faith. I do not understand why You have allowed my health challenges, but I trust You with my life. You created me, and You are still creating a work in and through me. Help me continue to live out Your plan for me. In Jesus's name, amen.

Embrace: My life may change to accommodate illness, but the God who never changes is still at work in my life.

Ponder: "Surrendering to the fear of greater illness will lead to hopelessness." Has the fear of greater illness created a defeated mindset in you? How can trusting God to work through your limitations help you be victorious despite them?

Worship: "Intentional (Album Version)" by Travis Greene

Break Through Pain

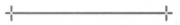

When you pass through the waters, I will be with you; and when you pass through the rivers, they will not sweep over you. When you walk through the fire, you will not be burned; the flames will not set you ablaze.

—*Isaiah 43:2*

Every part of me is affected when I am in a pain flare. Gravity presses on my burning muscles until they become heavy under the weight. I feel nothing but the burning and stinging and crushing that is my pain. My thoughts become scattered and lost in the fog that pain creates. Pain builds a wall that blocks my vision so that I lose sight of hope.

I may be cut off from the vigor of health, but I am never cut off from the Lord. Nothing—not trouble or hardship or affliction or pain or illness—can separate me from the love of Christ. His love helps me rise and more than conquer the tyranny of pain. It will not reign over me.

The Lord helps me rise even on the days when I cannot get out of bed. I rise up in faith through prayer. I rise into thanksgiving by singing praise songs. I rise out of despair by listening to gospel music. My prayers, my praise, and the singing voices of other believers converge to lift my spirit up, up, up out of my pain and into God's presence. His presence is peace. His presence is joy. His presence is comfort. Pain, with all its trickery and wiles, cannot enter this sacred space. The wall that pain built is shattered; my spirit is restored.

Pray: Dear God, You have promised that I am more than a conqueror through Jesus Christ. On the days when pain and illness have won the battle for my attention, help me remember Your love for me. Remind me that I am not alone. Thank You for giving me spiritual weapons against hopelessness and despair. Prayer and praise will break through the walls of hopelessness. Help me use Your Word to demolish anything that sets itself up to block my faith in You. Thank You for always giving me a way back to You. In Jesus's name, amen.

Embrace: Nothing—not trouble or hardship or affliction or pain or illness—can separate me from the love of Christ.

Practice: Write down one way you will rise up through praise during your next pain flare. Keep the note next to your bed so you will not forget.

Worship: "Praise Before My Breakthrough" by Bryan and Katie Torwalt

Can Sickness Make You Selfish?

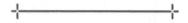

Those who live according to the flesh have their minds set on what the flesh desires; but those who live in accordance with the Spirit have their minds set on what the Spirit desires.
—Romans 8:5

Centering our lives around the challenges of illness can pull us off-balance like a rapidly spinning toy top that is knocked off its axis. Is it any surprise when we topple and run into those closest to us? Are you prone to impatience or selfishness when you do not feel well? I certainly am! But illness is not the cause of selfishness any more than it is the cause of impatience. The difficulties of living with illness propel us into survival mode, which can expose our human tendencies toward sin. Coming face-to-face with our selfishness, impatience, or ingratitude is difficult! But God does not condemn us; He forgives and transforms us so that we can ultimately experience greater freedom.

Take an honest inventory of your heart and your actions. Have you been short-tempered or impatient? Have you expected special treatment from others and become upset when you did not receive it? During illness, particularly extended illness, we need God's transforming and sustaining power to help us change any unhealthy patterns we have developed. If this has been an ongoing challenge for you, take heart. God's forgiveness is unending, and "there is now no condemnation for those who are in Christ Jesus" (Romans 8:1). Continue to seek God's help and ask for forgiveness from Him and others when frustration causes you to topple. When you make Jesus the central focus of your life, even the challenges of illness cannot pull you off your axis for long.

Pray: Dear God, please forgive me for the times when my illness or pain reveals an impatient spirit. Please show me if I am nurturing a bitter heart, and help me find freedom in forgiveness. Reveal any unhealthy patterns that I have developed, and show me how to break free from them. You are a God who delights in bringing freedom and peace. Thank You for Your mercies; they are new every day. Help me let go of anything that is keeping me from staying in step with Your Spirit. In Jesus's powerful name, amen.

Embrace: God's transforming and sustaining power can help me change unhealthy patterns.

Practice: Do you owe anyone an apology for being quick-tempered or selfish when you do not feel well? Make amends with them today. Simply say, "I'm sorry that I was not [patient, kind, and so on] when I was feeling poorly. Please forgive me." Illness is difficult for everyone in the family; the practice of making amends can lead to a stronger support system.

Worship: "Amazing Grace (My Chains Are Gone)" by Chris Tomlin

A Higher Purpose

*I want you to know, brothers and sisters, that what has happened
to me has actually served to advance the gospel.*
—*Philippians 1:12*

Paul wrote his letter to the Philippians while he was imprisoned. He could have written to tell them that the chains hurt, the prison food was terrible, and he was tired of persecution. Instead, he looked beyond his suffering and saw God's purpose in it. Paul rejoiced that his chains emboldened other believers to preach the gospel. He even rejoiced when those who wanted to stir up trouble for him preached the gospel. Paul never lost sight of his calling. He knew that God's purpose for his life could not be confined even during his confinement.

My cancer may have relapsed, but God's purpose for my life has never lapsed. He uses my infirmities to clarify my calling, as cancer has given me greater urgency and courage to tell others about Jesus. I do not want to be sick any more than Paul wanted to be in chains, but God uses the difficult realities of illness to help me develop an eternal perspective. If God has allowed cancer, chronic pain, or any other suffering, you can be sure it is not in vain. It will serve a purpose in your life and in the lives of those around you as you trust God and continue to serve Him in the midst of it.

Pray: Lord, help me learn from Paul's example. He never lost sight of his calling. Help me remember that Your purpose and calling for my life have not changed just because I have health issues. Open my eyes so I can see beyond my circumstances.

Thank You for the ways my illness opens up opportunities to share gospel hope. Give me the courage to tell others about You. In Jesus's name, amen.

Embrace: God's purpose for my life cannot be confined even when I am confined by illness.

Practice: Do you know the comfort, hope, and strength of faith in Jesus Christ? If not, ask God to lead you into truth and teach you how to have the hope of eternal life. See "You Can Know Jesus" in the Resources section for further information. If you already know Jesus, how have your health issues opened up opportunities to share gospel hope with others?

Worship: "Worth (Full Version)" by Anthony Brown and group therAPy

Lies like Snowflakes

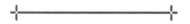

The Spirit God gave us does not make us timid, but gives us power, love and self-discipline.
—*2 Timothy 1:7*

Pain may have made me less mobile, but my fear of experiencing even more discomfort can completely immobilize me. Fear whispers lies that fall like gentle snowflakes, one after another. Fear tells me that only my vigilance will keep me safe from further suffering or harm. It cautions me that any movement might increase my pain. It warns me not to act, not to risk, not to make an effort that might make my life even more challenging. The lies stick together like snowflakes until a growing blanket of snow covers me. I become frozen by fear, so I decide to settle in and get used to the bitter cold.

But God speaks into this snowstorm. He asks, *Why are you afraid?* He reveals that my fear of suffering has kept me from living the life He has called me to lead. He reminds me not to love comfort more than I love Him. He instructs me not to be frozen by fear but to stand and follow Jesus. He tells me that He is always with me and will never forsake me. He calls me His beloved. His truth shines brightly, melting the icy fear that has made me brittle enough to snap. God's promises restore me. I am no longer frozen by fear; I am steeled by grace. I am strengthened by love. I am standing firm. And now I am ready to follow.

Pray: Dear God, You know my suffering. You understand the depths of my pain, and You have compassion for me. Please reveal the motivations of my heart. Forgive me if I long for relief from illness more than I long for You. Show me if physical comfort has become my idol. In the deepest recesses of my heart, please teach me how I can stand up under the burden of suffering. Melt my fears by the power of Your Word. Strengthen me. Restore me. Help me stand. In Jesus's powerful name, amen.

Embrace: The truth of God's Word melts my fears.

Ponder: What is one area in which you need to rely on the truth of God's Word rather than on how illness makes you feel?

Worship: "I'm Listening (Radio Version)" by Chris McClarney, featuring Hollyn

A Supernatural Companion

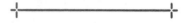

Who shall separate us from the love of Christ? Shall trouble or hardship or persecution or famine or nakedness or danger or sword? . . . No, in all these things we are more than conquerors through him who loved us.

—*Romans 8:35, 37*

Our lives are forever changed when we face severe health issues. Debilitating illness can threaten our employment, our relationships, and even our lives. It is no wonder insomnia often accompanies illness! As you lie awake at night hoping to drift into sleep, you might be too tired to close the door to unwelcome thoughts: *I should be enjoying life, not dealing with illness. My life is not worth anything if I have to live this way. I just cannot take it anymore.* When your mind is left unguarded by the toll of sleepless nights and unending pain, it is natural for these unwelcome visitors to become your companions through the sleepless night. But discouraging thoughts are a siren song, and they will always lead us into crashing waves of despair.

Turn away from the discouraging thoughts that are natural companions to suffering; instead, turn to a supernatural companion. Jesus is "a friend who sticks closer than a brother" (Proverbs 18:24). Nothing, not even illness or insomnia, will ever separate us from His love. I capture any unwelcome thoughts that tell me that my life is worthless (or worth less) because of pain or disease, and I surrender them to God. Then I invite the peace of Christ to guard my heart and mind throughout my sleepless nights. The greatest companion for my insomnia, pain, and suffering will always be my savior; by this, He proves He is saving me still.

Pray: Dear Jesus, You are the Companion of my soul. Thank You for loving me enough to save me from death; please continue to save me from the things that bring death to my spirit. Teach me how to recognize thoughts that are not from You so I can be quick to surrender them. Help me remember scriptures that bring hope, life, and peace, particularly when my suffering leaves me struggling to embrace Your goodness. Be my closest companion, Lord. I love You. In Your name, amen.

Embrace: I will turn away from the despairing thoughts that are natural companions to suffering; instead, I will turn to a supernatural companion.

Practice: On index cards, write down any negative thoughts that tend to arrive when you struggle with pain or illness. Find the common themes. For example, is discouragement a theme? If so, look for the word *encourage* on your Bible app or in your Bible's concordance. You can also search for "Bible verse, encourage" on the internet. Write down any verses that stand out to you. Counter each negative thought with truth from Scripture; keep the cards where you are most likely to see them. Read them aloud daily.

Worship: "What Can Separate You?" by Babbie Mason

Keep Reaching for Jesus

$\dashv$ ——————————— $\vdash$

> A woman was there who had been subject to bleeding for twelve years, but no one could heal her. She came up behind him and touched the edge of his cloak, and immediately her bleeding stopped.
>
> —*Luke 8:43–44*

Have you suffered from illness for years and years? Have you gone from doctor to doctor, from surgery to surgery, from medical bill to medical bill? If so, you can relate to the biblical account of the woman who reached out to touch Jesus's cloak. According to Levitical law, her condition made her unclean, so if anyone touched her, they would become unclean as well. Imagine her desperation as she pushed into the crowd, being careful not to transfer her unclean state. Gently, almost imperceptibly, she reached out to touch the edge of Jesus's garment and was immediately healed. Jesus could have let her quietly slip back into the crowd, back to the judgment-filled whispers about why she had been afflicted. But He loved her too much to let her sneak away in fear, alone and unnoticed.

"Who touched me?" Jesus asked. "Someone touched me; I know that power has gone out from me" (Luke 8:45–46). The Lord who created her, the God who knew every single hair on her head, surely knew the identity of the woman He had healed. But He was about to restore more than her health. This woman had suffered in every conceivable way: loss of health, loss of finances, loss of standing in the community. Perhaps even loss of faith, until now. Jesus loved her so much that He publicly restored her by saying, "Daughter, your faith has healed you. Go in peace" (verse 48). She came to Jesus for physical healing, but she left with so much more.

Pray: Dear Jesus, You have taken away my unclean state by forgiving my sins, and my faith in You has restored me to spiritual wholeness. I will not take this healing and return to my old way of life; I will continue to follow You. You have not changed; You still have the power to heal me. Until that time, Your power is made perfect in my weakness. Help me experience and recognize Your power in my life today, Lord. In Your name I pray. Amen.

Embrace: When I reach out to Jesus, He gives me more than I ever hoped to find.

Ponder: Jesus's power is made manifest according to His purposes for our lives. The Lord told the apostle Paul, "My grace is sufficient for you, for my power is made perfect in weakness" (2 Corinthians 12:9). Do you pray for Jesus's sustaining power as much as you pray for His healing power? Why or why not?

Worship: "He Touched Me" by Joey + Rory

Hidden Fruit Is Still Fruit

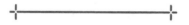

I am the vine; you are the branches. If you remain in me and
I in you, you will bear much fruit; apart from me you can do
nothing.

—*John 15:5*

I have not been very fruitful in good works since illness has isolated
me, so I asked God where I should be fruitful. He spoke to my
spirit and said, *Sometimes fruit lies close to the vine.* Fruit that is nestled
against the vine may not be readily noticed, but it is still fruit. Even
the sweetest grapes can be concealed. These devotionals are my hidden fruit; I write them while I am homebound and clinging tightly to
Jesus. I often wonder how God will use this fruit. Will it be consumed
by a single soul and bring a bit of refreshment to that one person, or
will it be mixed with other fruit into preserves that sweeten the lives
of many?

Often, sharp rocks are found in the soil of areas notable for producing wonderful grapes. It seems that the stones absorb heat during the day, which is released at night. The rocks help keep the soil at
the right temperature for the best grapes to grow. I do not like the
rocks that sharpen the soil of my life. Disease, suffering, and disappointment crowd my life to the point that sometimes I feel incapable
of producing any fruit at all. But the warmth of God's life-giving
presence soaks into every difficulty and enables me to bear the best
fruit. These painful rocks have a purpose. God uses all my circumstances to create the best growing conditions. Being homebound by
illness allows me the opportunity to embrace my proximity to the
vine. It turns out that hidden fruit is hidden from only the world.
God sees the fruit I bear while I bear up under suffering.

Pray: Dear Lord, it is so difficult to be isolated by illness. Help me cling to You for support. Difficulties can make me seem barren, but You promise that I will never be fruitless when I remain in You. May Your presence transform the hard things, even the sharp pain and crushing illness, into opportunity for abundant growth. May You be glorified and honored by the fruit I produce during this season. I love You, Lord. In Your name, amen.

Embrace: The warmth of God's life-giving presence soaks into every difficulty and enables me to bear the best fruit.

Ponder: How has illness isolated you or caused you to feel fruitless? What is the way to continue to have a life that produces something beautiful? (Hint: Reread John 15:5.)

Worship: "Full Attention" by Jeremy Riddle

Stormy Seas and Turbulent Treetops

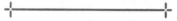

When he saw the wind, he was afraid and, beginning to sink, cried out, "Lord, save me!" Immediately Jesus reached out his hand and caught him. "You of little faith," he said, "why did you doubt?" And when they climbed into the boat, the wind died down.

—*Matthew 14:30–32*

There is a beautiful yellow bird on the tree branch outside my window. The branch bends and sways in the strong wind, but that stubborn bird holds on through it all. I am amazed that it doesn't fly away or glide to the ground, where it won't be blown to and fro. Perhaps it is having fun up there in its domain of wind and leaves and sky. Perhaps it is patiently waiting out the storm on this unpredictable roller-coaster ride of heights and dips. Or perhaps it is just holding on with everything God gave it.

That bird doesn't ever slip. It doesn't panic or look to the other birds to see how they handle the blustery wind. It just holds tightly until something else comes its way: a better perch, a tasty insect, or the call of another creature. The tiny bird doesn't wonder why it is all alone on that branch or if the winds will ever die down. It just does what it is equipped to do. With lightweight tail feathers for balance and claws to grasp even the smallest branch, the bird is prepared to handle life in the treetops, winds and all.

You also are equipped to handle storms, because God has given you everything you need in Christ. Whatever the Lord has allowed for you—whatever job, family, neighborhood, pain, or illness—He will help you and empower you. You are His most precious creation. Since He cares for the birds of the air, how much more will He care for you? So hold tightly to Him by praying and believing His Word. Trust that He is in charge of the winds that blow. He is still God. He is still good. You can trust Him to help you in the midst of any storm.

Pray: Dear God, thank You that You are with me in every storm. You give me all I need: strength when I am weary, hope when I am discouraged, and endurance when I feel like giving up. Turn my eyes back to You when I start to compare my storm with someone else's. If I fall, let it be into Your arms. Thank You for never leaving me. Please help me by the power of Your Holy Spirit. In Jesus's name, amen.

Embrace: Jesus equips me with all I need to endure the storms in my life.

Ponder: Birds do not look around to see how other creatures are handling blustery winds. When you are experiencing trials, do you ever compare your life or ability to cope with that of others? Does this help or hinder your faith in God's provision for you?

Worship: "Not Afraid" by Jesus Culture, featuring Kim Walker-Smith

Sharing in His Suffering

Since we are his children, we are his heirs. In fact, together with Christ we are heirs of God's glory. But if we are to share his glory, we must also share his suffering.

—*Romans 8:17, NLT*

The burning of complex regional pain syndrome (CRPS) often feels like a garment of flames grafting itself into my skin. There are times when I no longer seem to know the difference between myself and my pain. All of me feels like pain; the bones crush, and the fires rage until I am almost lost in the heat. But I am not lost. Jesus is in the fire alongside me. He understands the depths of my pain; I see the evidence in His own scarred hands. His life becomes more real to me when His suffering is not just something I ponder but something I experience more deeply because of my own pain. If I am to follow Him, then I must walk as He did. Like Jesus, I plead with God to take this cup from me. Since the cup remains, I will trust Him as I sip from it.

One day God will bind it all together: all the pain, all the sorrows, and all the tears along with all of faith's perseverance, all of hope's steadfastness, all of love's faithfulness. He will shake them together in His hands, sift them through fingers of righteousness, and blow away the suffering until nothing remains that is not of Him. Then He will usher me into the life that is truly life. I will give up this crown of pain with these thorns of suffering, just as Jesus did, trading them for the crown of life He promised to those who endure. And I will embrace Him with joy.

Pray: Lord, sometimes the agony of pain and illness seems like it will never end. But You promise that there will be an end to all these things; there will be a new beginning, and with it will come complete restoration. Thank You that I can rest in that knowledge today. Give me the comfort that comes from remembering that I must share in Your suffering to one day share in Your glory. Give me the perseverance and perspective I need to endure everything that I face today. In Your mighty name I pray. Amen.

Embrace: Jesus understands the depths of my pain; I see the evidence in His own scarred hands.

Ponder: How do you share in Christ's suffering right now? In what ways does suffering draw you closer to the One who suffered for you?

Worship: "You Get the Glory" by Jonathan Traylor

God Will Never Fail Me

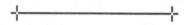

My health may fail, and my spirit may grow weak, but God remains the strength of my heart; he is mine forever.
—*Psalm 73:26, NLT*

Do you feel as though you cannot take any more illness or pain? Have you ever considered ways to take your life, as a means to end your pain? Friend, those thoughts may appear to help you escape suffering, but what they really show is that your heart is losing hope. Do not let a weary heart determine your steps! Let your actions be guided by wisdom, not captured and dragged away by hopelessness. Commit all your ways to God. Confess any thoughts that lead away from life and truth.

Do not keep thoughts of harming yourself a secret. Like seeds, they can germinate and grow when hidden in the soil of your mind. Instead, expose them to the light by telling someone. Speak with a counselor, pastor, doctor, or wise family member if you are struggling. Ask a friend or someone from church to pray with you. A hopeless heart steals your strength, so ask God to strengthen your spirit.

The Lord will sustain you moment by moment during illness. He will never fail you or abandon you, so don't give up. You will look back on this season of life with amazement at God's provision. Hold on to His promises, and when your strength fails, be upheld by the Lord's love for you. There is no one else just like you, occupying your exact place in our world. I am glad you are here; this world is a better place with you in it.

Pray: Dear God, illness and pain have led me into hopelessness. Help me guard my spirit against thoughts that steal my hope. Open my eyes so I can recognize when I entertain thoughts that lead to a pity party. Someone always gets hurt at that kind of party, and it is usually me. Build up a support system for me, and help me reach out to others. Protect my heart with gratitude that ignites joy. Restore me and give me an obedient heart. I rest in Your abiding love for me. You have a good plan for my life. In Jesus's name, amen.

Embrace: I will not allow a weary heart to determine my actions.

Practice: Please get help if you are experiencing thoughts of self-harm. Speak with a trusted pastor, counselor, or family member. See the Resources section for emergency-hotline numbers.

Worship: "You Belong Here" by Mike Donehey

Hope for More

We who have fled to take hold of the hope set before us may be greatly encouraged. We have this hope as an anchor for the soul, firm and secure.

—*Hebrews 6:18–19*

When I was in my early twenties, I hoped to become a kindergarten teacher and have children of my own one day. I became a teacher, albeit for first grade instead of kindergarten, and I was blessed with children. I no longer hope for those things, because a hope fulfilled is no longer a hope: "Hope that is seen is no hope at all. Who hopes for what they already have? But if we hope for what we do not yet have, we wait for it patiently" (Romans 8:24–25).

Have any of your hopes been fulfilled? What new desires have taken their place? Perhaps you yearn for the healing that seems out of reach. Allowing all your hope to rest on something that may or may not happen can lead to a crisis of faith. God placed the desire for wholeness and healing within us to point us toward wholeness in Christ and true healing that lasts for eternity. Your desire for healing can lead you to greater faith as you discover the true hope of an eternal perspective. God gives us far more than this world can offer. He can miraculously heal us, and we pray for this, but eternal healing is our only assured hope. Salvation promises bodily restoration, resurrection, and eternal life in heaven. One day we will be *fully* healed, and until that time, God "has given us everything we need for a godly life through our knowledge of him" (2 Peter 1:3). Wait patiently for Him to fulfill all His promises to you. Lean into the true hope we have in Christ; faith endures when you anchor it to hope that is sure.

Pray: Dear God, You are all-knowing, so You know all my hopes. Your Word tells me to delight myself in You and You will fulfill my heart's desires. Teach me to delight completely in You so I will be content with Your plans for my life. Hear my prayers for healing, and give me patience to wait for Your timing. May my desire for healing lead me to the assurance of eternal healing. In Jesus's name, amen.

Embrace: God placed the desire for wholeness and healing within me to point me toward true healing in Christ that lasts for eternity.

Ponder: Job was a man who lived before Jesus was born. He greatly hoped for healing. He was eventually healed, but in the midst of his agony, he said, "Oh, that I might have my request, that God would grant what I hope for. . . . What strength do I have, that I should still hope? What prospects, that I should be patient?" (Job 6:8, 11). How does faith give you the strength to hope? How does the prospect of future restoration help you wait patiently for healing?

Worship: "I Will Rise" by Chris Tomlin

Pain Cannot Take Everything

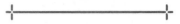

Praise be to the God and Father of our Lord Jesus Christ, who has blessed us in the heavenly realms with every spiritual blessing in Christ.

—Ephesians 1:3

Those of us with debilitating chronic pain are not joining teams, wearing ribbons, or running races to raise awareness of our illness. We cannot regularly attend church or Bible studies even on the days when we can manage to get out of bed; pain prevents us from sitting in a chair for hours at a time. We are often unable to volunteer for things that give us joy and a sense of purpose. We become the invisible, missed for a few days or weeks, then seemingly forgotten. We may even be homebound—but we are still here. We are still alive, and we feel the pain to prove it.

Pain robs us of much; it is a thief at heart. But it can never take away the hope, inner strength, and joy that are ours through Jesus Christ. The flesh may make us weak, but the Holy Spirit gives us strength to endure through every moment. One day our war with pain will end and our steadfast faith will be rewarded. We can soldier on with the knowledge that our hope—our *true* hope—is not lost. We may never live a pain-free life on this earth, but living an abundant life in the Spirit makes us truly free.

Pray: Dear Lord, I grieve the things that illness and pain have taken from me. You came to restore and redeem my life for eternity; give me patient hope for my redemption. Help me see beyond my present circumstances; open the eyes of my heart to know the fullness of healing and restoration that is mine in You.

Use my temporary afflictions to transform me, doing a thorough work so I will be mature and complete, lacking nothing. Fill me with Your Holy Spirit, and give me all I need in order to endure with patient hope. In Your name, amen.

Embrace: I may never live a pain-free life on this earth, but living an abundant life in the Spirit makes me truly free.

Ponder: People often mistake Jesus's promise of abundant life for an assurance of a life free from hardship; they get discouraged when life becomes difficult. How can believing this falsehood lead to crises of faith? In what ways does truly abundant spiritual life help us persevere with joy despite difficulties?

Worship: "It Is Well with My Soul" by Matt Redman

The Sacred Space

God is our refuge and strength, an ever-present help in trouble.
—*Psalm 46:1*

Severe chronic pain has taught me the power and fullness of the presence of Jesus. It is one thing to notice a firefighter on the way to a fire; it is another thing entirely to see that firefighter coming to your rescue when your home is aflame. At times, pain's burning embers join the fuel of fatigue and illness, exploding into a fire so hot I am overcome. It is not enough that my body feels the force of its heat; I suffocate in the fumes of self-pity and despair that travel with it. And just like that, pain transforms the fresh air of peace and contentment into toxic smoke that blankets me like a veil. Pain clouds my mind and robs my sight; it wants all of me. Disoriented, I no longer know the way of escape.

I would be utterly consumed if not for the Lord. I cry out to Him, desperately seeking Him amid the flames until He is all I see. My savior enters the raging fires of pain, and His comfort gives me a space of refuge. He holds me so close to His heart that even the smoke cannot come between us. The fire still rages, but now I can breathe. I inhale His strength, love, and comfort. I exhale my fear, desolation, and hopelessness. I am safe in this sacred space.

Pray: Lord, today the fires of illness are raging in my body. Come to my rescue. Enter my suffering, fill me with the living water of Your Spirit, and saturate me with the truth of Your

Word. No blaze can consume me when I am filled to overflowing with Your living water. May I experience Your great love and powerful strength until I have no room for anything but You. Thank You for being my refuge from the fires of pain and suffering. In Your name, amen.

Embrace: Jesus's comfort gives me a space of refuge from the fires of affliction.

Ponder: What stood out to you as you read my account of Jesus's help during a pain flare? How does His comfort give us refuge from suffering?

Worship: "Closer" by Maverick City Music, featuring Brandon Lake

Pain and Punishment

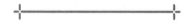

It is for freedom that Christ has set us free. Stand firm, then, and
do not let yourselves be burdened again by a yoke of slavery.
—*Galatians 5:1*

When you are having a bad day with illness, do you ever ask
yourself, *What did I do to trigger my pain or fatigue? Was it some-*
thing I ate? Was I too active? Those questions create a burden of guilt
because they make your health challenges seem like your fault. They
may even expose an underlying belief that your disease is caused by a
character defect instead of a health defect. I began to notice that I felt
overwhelmingly responsible when I experienced insomnia during a
pain flare, as if sheer willpower could take away my pain and make
me fall asleep. My misplaced guilt had deep roots: It developed in
childhood.

Many people with chronic pain and serious health issues have experienced childhood trauma.[3] My own childhood was marked by
physical abuse. Children typically believe the abuse is their fault, so I
tried to become "good enough" to avoid having pain inflicted on me.
My childlike effort was really an attempt at controlling the unpredictable and frightening behavior of someone I loved. Now when I
have pain, I feel just like that little girl who thought she did something to cause it. Although my disease is also unpredictable and
frightening, I cannot be "good enough" to make it stop. It is futile to
think that way.

Your childhood may have been similarly marked by trauma. You
may have even heard people say, "The body keeps score." The theory

is that childhood trauma causes harmful changes to our minds and bodies that can persist through adulthood. When I learned this concept, I felt trapped, as though I would never escape my childhood harm. But our minds and bodies are fearfully and wonderfully created by the God who heals. You cannot change the past, but you can invite Him to heal your present connection to it. He can help you speak of your sorrows, share your burdens, and shake off your shackles of unforgiveness. Are you familiar with the saying "Refusing to forgive is like drinking poison and expecting the other person to die"? Forgiveness sets you free from the pain that abuse ignited in your spirit. It is the greatest gift you can give yourself.

Your childhood may have taught you that you were responsible for the things that hurt you. If so, pay attention to how this underlying false belief shapes your thoughts about living with illness. Do you feel responsible when you cannot control your health issues? Do you feel crushing guilt when your pain flares, your mind is muddled by brain fog, or your fatigue keeps you from being active? Accepting the additional weight of false guilt makes the burden of illness feel unbearable. "It is for freedom that Christ has set us free" (Galatians 5:1); let's live in freedom by rejecting any false beliefs that were created by past trauma.

Pray: God, thank You for setting me free from everything that has the power to harm me. You are my healer and my provider; You lead me in paths of healing righteousness for Your name's sake. Shed light on the beliefs that hinder my freedom. Forgive me for thinking that I am wholly responsible for my health issues; release me from the burden of false guilt. Please help me forgive anyone who has harmed me. I trust You to hold them accountable. I will no longer allow bitterness or anger to trick me into thinking it holds someone accountable. Thank You for the freedom of forgiveness. In Jesus's name, amen.

Embrace: I will live in freedom by rejecting any false beliefs that were created by past trauma.

Practice: God loved you enough to take the full punishment for sin. Your pain is not a punishment, even when it feels like one. Read Isaiah 53:5. Who paid the price and took the complete punishment for sin? Also read Lamentations 3:32–33. What do these verses tell you about God's compassion for you?

Worship: "No Longer Slaves (Radio Remix)" by Jonathan David Helser and Melissa Helser

A Greeting Card for Chronic Illness

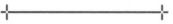

Singing cheerful songs to a person with a heavy heart is like taking someone's coat in cold weather or pouring vinegar in a wound.

—*Proverbs 25:20, NLT*

I wrote the "greeting card" below after receiving a well-intentioned but poorly-thought-out card from a friend. It advised me to dance through difficulties during a time when I could not even walk without assistance. This is the greeting card that I would have liked to have received during that painful season:

Healthy people often send
Greeting cards containing
Verses that admonish you,
"Smile! It will soon stop raining."

I could send you something quaint
With pretty words or rhyme—
Something to convey the message
"You will be 'just fine.'"

But instead of lofty sentiment
Arriving in pretty verse,
Alluding to your illness,
Saying it won't get worse,

I come to meet you where you are
In that lonely place of pain,

Knowing that your reality is
Rain and Rain and Rain and Rain
And Rain.

Pray: Dear Lord, thank You for meeting me exactly where I am. You are the only one who truly understands my suffering. Help me be patient with people when their attempts to cheer me up leave me feeling worse. Give me compassion for them; help them have the same for me. Shelter me with Your presence during every rainstorm. Thank You for Your heart of compassion for me, Lord. In Your name, amen.

Embrace: I will seek shelter in the Lord during the rainy seasons of my life.

Practice: Jesus is a friend who meets us in our lonely place of pain. He also uses the church to do His work. Are you connected with another believer who can support you during the difficulties of chronic illness? If not, call your local church and ask to be connected with someone. See "You Can Know Jesus" in the Resources section to find a Bible-believing church near you.

Worship: "Praise You in This Storm" by Casting Crowns

Good Medicine

A cheerful heart is good medicine, but a crushed spirit dries up the bones.

—*Proverbs 17:22*

I t is one thing to live with a broken body; it is another thing altogether to live with a broken body and a devastated spirit. Does your spirit feel such sorrow that you wonder how you will ever recover? You might feel like the prophet Habakkuk, who described the physical manifestations of his crushed spirit: "My heart pounded, my lips quivered at the sound; decay crept into my bones, and my legs trembled" (Habakkuk 3:16). Nothing crushes a spirit more than fear that gives rise to hopelessness. The prophet Jeremiah spoke of the anguish of a crushed spirit when he said, "I remember my affliction and my wandering, the bitterness and the gall. I well remember them, and my soul is downcast within me" (Lamentations 3:19–20).

How do you heal a crushed spirit and downcast soul? Both Habakkuk and Jeremiah confessed fear, hopelessness, and sorrow, then spoke one word that turned everything around. What is the one word that began the healing process? *Yet.* Habakkuk followed his fears with "*Yet* I will wait patiently. . . . *Yet* I will rejoice in the LORD, I will be joyful in God my Savior" (Habakkuk 3:16, 18, emphasis added). Jeremiah also knew the power of moving beyond pain by saying, "*Yet* this I call to mind and therefore I have hope: Because of the LORD's great love we are not consumed, for his compassions never fail" (Lamentations 3:21–22, emphasis added).

A crushed spirit can be restored. Begin the healing process by voicing your complaint to God in prayer. Rejoice in the Lord by giving thanks. Remember that a cheerful heart is good medicine that helps your spirit endure illness. You may be living with tremendous challenges, *yet* you will always have reason to rejoice in the unchanging goodness of the Lord.

Pray: Dear Lord, I need a strong spirit to endure illness; help me recognize when my spirit is crushed. Thank You that You give me a remedy for healing. I praise You for keeping my spirit strong when I am overcome by pain or illness. I am suffering, *yet* I will choose to rejoice in Your goodness. Thank You that You never leave me or forsake me. I love You, Lord. Amen.

Embrace: A cheerful heart is good medicine that helps my spirit endure illness.

Practice: The Old Testament book of Lamentations is filled with laments, or expressions of sorrow. Write your own lament, and then follow it with *yet* and your declarations of God's goodness. The things you write after the word *yet* will become a bridge from suffering into greater faith.

Worship: "Though You Slay Me" by Shane & Shane

Disappointed or Delighted?

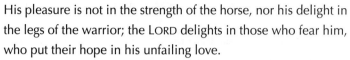

His pleasure is not in the strength of the horse, nor his delight in
the legs of the warrior; the LORD delights in those who fear him,
who put their hope in his unfailing love.
—*Psalm 147:10–11*

D o you feel frustrated with yourself on those days when you cannot manage to push past your health challenges? I used to
think that God was disappointed with me when pain kept me from
getting out of bed. It is a mistake to project our feelings onto other
people, but it is downright dangerous when we attribute our feelings
to God. My disappointment that illness had affected my activities
did not mean God was disappointed in me.

Have you ever felt as though you are a disappointment to God
because you cannot serve Him in the ways you used to when you were
healthy? It is a trap of the worst kind to believe that your limitations
make you a disappointment to your loving Father. He knows your
capabilities and frailties because He is your creator. He saw you and
loved you even before your body had taken shape in the womb. Jesus
became flesh and endured suffering, so He understands the demands
of hurting flesh. Remember that your flesh may fail but God's unconditional love for you never will.

Living with illness is so difficult that it often brings us to our
knees. Whether you can actually kneel or not, let those days remind
you of your need to bow your thoughts to God in prayer. You create
a place of peace in your war with illness when you surrender your
frustrations to God. Confess any anger or impatience that the difficulties of disease have stirred up within you, and then receive God's
forgiveness and loving compassion. He delights in you when you ac-

knowledge Him and continue to hope in the unfailing love that He gives us through Jesus Christ. You may not have been able to get out of bed today. You may feel disappointed with yourself. But your weaknesses and limitations will never diminish God's love for you.

Pray: Dear God, please help me accept Your grace and compassion when my illness makes it difficult to do the good things I would like to do. Enable my heart to trust Your plan for me right now. I know that You do not delight in my physical abilities but You delight in those who fear You and put their hope in Your unfailing love. Thank You that even when my body fails, Your loving-kindness never does. Give me peace as I rest in Your love for me today. In Jesus's name, amen.

Embrace: My flesh may fail, but God's unconditional love for me never will.

Ponder: Have you ever worried that God is disappointed in you because of your limitations? How does placing your hope in His unconditional love release you from this burden?

Worship: "I Am Loved" by Mack Brock

Hearing the News

†————————————†

You will keep in perfect peace those whose minds are steadfast,
because they trust in you.
—Isaiah 26:3

I was already in pre-op when my doctor received my biopsy results, just as he was about to perform an additional surgery on me. He informed me that I had two forms of advanced-stage lymphoma and that one was aggressive. Although I was surprised, I knew that my cancer was not a surprise to God. He had faithfully helped me throughout years of debilitating illness, and I knew He would continue to help me through cancer. Healing would arrive on earth or in heaven, but either way I would be healed. My doctor looked devastated by the news he had to deliver, so I shared my faith with him.

I do not recall exactly what I said that day, but I do remember the nurse who overheard the entire encounter. He pulled me aside later and said, "As long as I live, I will never forget how you responded to the news of your cancer. I have witnessed many people get that news and have never seen someone respond with so much faith and peace." My memory of that day is marked not by fear but by the beautiful blessing of making an impact by simply sharing stored-up truth. Nothing, not even cancer, can move us when we are firmly convinced of God's sovereignty and loving care. Trusting a dependable God during a difficult diagnosis is the pathway to peace.

Pray: Dear God, thank You that I can depend on You even
during a difficult diagnosis. My health issues may change,
but You are the God who never changes. You are always trust-

worthy. Please help me store up Your Word in my heart and mind so I will overflow with faith. Thank You that prayer and thanksgiving lead to peace that guards my heart and mind. Help me have steadfast trust that keeps me in perfect peace. In Jesus's name, amen.

Embrace: Trusting a dependable God during a difficult diagnosis is the pathway to peace.

Ponder: Where do you turn to find peace during difficult times? Do you try to manufacture your own peace, or do you trust God and receive His peace?

Worship: "I Will Trust My Saviour Jesus" by CityAlight

Jesus Is My Right-Hand Man

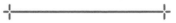

I keep my eyes always on the LORD. With him at my right hand,
I will not be shaken. Therefore my heart is glad and my tongue
rejoices; my body also will rest secure.
> —*Psalm 16:8–9*

C an you recall a time when your illness severely limited your ability to function? An accident to my left hand triggered complex
regional pain syndrome (CRPS), a debilitatingly painful disease that
limits limb function. I began to rely on my right hand for daily tasks,
but this is harder than it sounds, because I am left-handed. One day
I tried to open my heavy bedroom curtains with my right hand, but
it was also too frozen by stiffness and pain to grasp the drapery cord.
As it so often does, CRPS had spread to my opposite limb. The disease had already reached my feet, so I was crushed by the realization
that it now affected all my limbs.

I inwardly panicked and thought, *Lord, I cannot do this. How will I
live my life without the full use of both hands?* Immediately, I sensed the
Lord's answer to my unspoken question: *I will be with you along the
way, and we will meet each challenge together.* Receiving God's comfort
gave me strength to steel myself against the frustration and helpless-
ness of self-pity. Truth transformed my thinking, so I was able to
declare, *All right, Lord. I have physical limitations today, but it is okay because You are with me and will help me each step of the way.*

Do you recall a time when you were also confronted by the harsh
realities of life with illness? Telling yourself the truth about God's
faithfulness will dispel fears about your future. We can more easily
accept our limitations when we remember that God is not limited by
anything. He is by your side and will help you through the difficulties

of illness. Your limitations will never limit God's ability or willingness to help you through them.

Pray: Lord, sometimes my health makes the daily tasks of life so difficult. Remind me when I struggle that You are my helper. Thank You that You are always with me and will never leave my side. I do not need to panic and try to control everything that affects me, because You keep watch over all that concerns me. Thank You that everything You allow in my life will ultimately work together to bring about Your best for me. In Your name, amen.

Embrace: My limitations will never limit God's ability or willingness to help me through them.

Ponder: How can remembering that you are equipped by God's presence protect you from fear and self-pity?

Worship: "I Have This Hope" by Tenth Avenue North

My Daily Victory

Blessed is the one who perseveres under trial because, having stood the test, that person will receive the crown of life that the Lord has promised to those who love him.

—James 1:12

Have you ever felt such deep pain and exhaustion that getting out of bed every morning feels like fighting a battle? Years ago, I attempted to describe this battle in my journal, so I personified pain and exhaustion as actual enemies. You might be able to relate to my story:

Pain is the first thing to greet me every morning; it breaks into my dreams and clamors for all my attention. As I struggle to wake, I remember that Exhaustion is Pain's closest companion. It is difficult to fight Pain, but the battle against Exhaustion is more easily won, and Wakefulness triumphs. Sometimes I wish to forfeit the fight with Exhaustion and drift back into a sea of sweet sleep, unawake and unaware that Pain is lurking near. But I must press on and fight the battle to get up every morning.

Pain and Exhaustion are tenacious foes, but I have a secret weapon. First, I ask God to fill me with His Spirit. Then I pray for the strength to press through pain. I refuse to be dismayed if I need to lie down after taking my morning shower. Instead, I will praise God that I was able to shower. If I am too weak or in too much pain to get out of bed, then I will lie there and thank Him for my blessings. Gratitude will guard my reservoir of strength so I can persevere through my health challenges.

The Holy Spirit indwells me and encourages me to continue the fight and live in such a way that pain does not become my god. I will not bow to it or let it rule over me. The Lord strengthens my spirit to stand firm amid this daily battle. He always leads me to victory, so I am determined to persevere.

Pray: Dear Jesus, You know the battles I face, and You understand because You faced them first. You suffered great pain on the cross, but You stayed on it. You did not give up or give in because it was difficult. I believe in You, so Your Spirit lives in me. Help me rely on Your Spirit to strengthen and encourage me. Give me all I need in order to persevere today. In Your name, amen.

Embrace: Gratitude will guard my reservoir of strength so I can persevere through my health challenges.

Ponder: How does strengthening your spirit help you live with physical pain without allowing it to rule over you? What is one way that you are taking care of your spirit right now so you can persevere?

Worship: "No Weapon" by Fred Hammond and Radical for Christ

Taking Shelter

I cry to you, LORD; I say, "You are my refuge, my portion in the land of the living." Listen to my cry, for I am in desperate need; rescue me from those who pursue me, for they are too strong for me.

—*Psalm 142:5–6*

In the Old Testament book of Numbers, God commanded the Levite priests to set aside six of their towns as cities of refuge (see 35:6–15). These places of shelter were designed to harbor people who had accidentally killed someone; there they would be kept safe from anyone seeking to avenge the death. The roads leading to these cities of refuge were to be a smooth and easily maneuvered path to safety; clearly marked signs may have even pointed the way there. God ensured that traveling to shelter would not be difficult, since those who needed protection often had to quickly escape a pursuer.

Health issues are relentless pursuers; they attack when we least expect. But Jesus already paved the way to refuge. Illness and death may try to pursue us, but His goodness and mercy catch us first. No matter what you are facing—surgeries, cancer treatments, unrelenting pain, being homebound—you will not be overcome by these adversaries when you seek refuge in God. He has given you eternal shelter. You are safe.

Pray: Dear God, You are my refuge and strength. Shelter me from anything that might harm me. Preserve my life according to Your Word. Thank You that Jesus paved the difficult path to sanctuary so my hope of salvation is secure. Guard me from temptation, and help me run directly to You when I am in need.

Thank You for saving me from all that pursues me and for giving me eternal refuge from death. In Jesus's name, amen.

Embrace: I have eternal refuge because Jesus already paved the way to shelter.

Ponder: The psalmist King David declared, "Surely goodness and mercy and unfailing love shall follow me all the days of my life, and I shall dwell forever [throughout all my days] in the house and in the presence of the Lord" (Psalm 23:6, AMP). Have you ever felt as though you are being pursued by illness? If so, how does it change your mindset to picture God's goodness, mercy, and love pursuing you instead?

Worship: "The Name of Jesus" by Chris Tomlin

The Burden of Offense

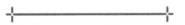

Above all, have fervent and unfailing love for one another, because love covers a multitude of sins [it overlooks unkindness and unselfishly seeks the best for others].
—*1 Peter 4:8, AMP*

If you have not been offended by others during your illness, either you have not been listening to them or you have not been sick for very long! From doctors making belittling comments to friends misunderstanding the ways your illness affects your life, there are plenty of opportunities to take offense. But unless we want to sit around in a state of perpetual anger, we must learn to move past perceived slights. Do you want to leave the anger of offense and move on toward peace? It is easier said than done, but it is possible. God gave us a way. When we choose to forgive, we release the burden of offense back to the One who bears our burdens.

Living with illness is hard enough; I do not want anything else to weigh me down in this life, including the burden of offense. The author of Ecclesiastes exhorted, "Do not be quickly provoked in your spirit, for anger resides in the lap of fools" (7:9). I stop allowing anger to crawl into my lap when I take a spiritual stand in the power that Jesus Christ died to give me. I will move unhindered down the path of forgiveness, allowing petty provocations to provoke me to greater peace.

Pray: Dear Lord, forgive me when I am easily provoked.
It hurts me when I perceive a lack of compassion toward me.
When I am in pain or struggling with illness, even a tiny slight
can cut deeply. Please give me Your perspective. Help me think

the best of others. Fill my heart with the love that triumphs over an unforgiving spirit. Lead me down the path of forgiveness. I choose to walk with You today. In Your name, amen.

Embrace: I will allow petty provocations to provoke me to greater peace.

Ponder: What provocations have you nurtured by allowing them to crawl into your lap and stay close to you? What steps will you take to stand, brush them off, and move past them today?

Worship: "Forgiveness" by Matthew West

Perseverance Is Patient

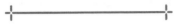

You have carefully followed my doctrine, manner of life, purpose, faith, longsuffering, love, perseverance, persecutions, afflictions. . . . And out of them all the Lord delivered me.
—2 Timothy 3:10–11, NKJV

Years ago, as a young Christian, I believed that a blessed life meant freedom from trials. It was wishful thinking, not biblical thinking, because I had resolutely ignored the many Scripture verses warning that faithful believers will undergo painful trials. I am not alone in this; many of us want our faith in God to ensure that our earthly lives will be free from suffering. Many of us have read a Bible verse about long-suffering and thought, *Anything but that, Lord,* instead of recognizing it as a beautiful gift of patience that equips us to endure trials. We miss out on true blessing when we fail to embrace every part of God's Word as truth that sustains us.

Now, many hardships later, I realize that God is sovereign over all things in my life, including my health struggles. The presence of God's blessing does not mean the absence of pain and suffering. When I submit to Him in the midst of my illness, looking to Him for hope and strength, He gives me all I need to endure it. *Long-suffering* is no longer a term I fear; I joyfully embrace this blessing as a gift of patience that enables me to persevere through any hardship.

Pray: God, You know all things, so You know that I would like to be delivered from all sickness, pain, and hardship. Please help me stay rooted in You so I may bear the fruit of long-suffering, which gives me the strength to endure. Teach me to trust You as I wait patiently for deliverance from these hardships. Hold me close to Your heart, for I am so weary. Open my eyes so I may recognize all the ways You have equipped me to run the race You have appointed for me. I rejoice in You today. In Jesus's name, amen.

Embrace: Long-suffering is a gift of patience that enables me to persevere through any hardship.

Ponder: "The presence of God's blessing does not mean the absence of pain and suffering." Do you believe this to be true? Which scriptures can you find to support your belief?

Worship: "While I Wait" by Lincoln Brewster

Let There Be Life

Even when we are weighed down with troubles, it is for your comfort and salvation! For when we ourselves are comforted, we will certainly comfort you. Then you can patiently endure the same things we suffer.

—*2 Corinthians 1:6, NLT*

A re you inspired by stories of people who have persevered despite tremendous challenges? I greatly admire people such as Corrie ten Boom, Amy Carmichael, and Joni Eareckson Tada, who exemplify courage, faith, and tenacity in the face of adversity. God equipped them to fulfill their callings even amid soul-crushing circumstances. Significant ministries arose out of their considerable suffering.

Out of horrific Nazi brutality came the beauty of Corrie ten Boom's forgiveness and message of Christ's love.

Out of her many health struggles, Amy Carmichael was led to missions in India, where she devoted her life to helping orphaned children, sharing the gospel, and writing books that still inspire.

Out of lost mobility, Joni Eareckson Tada began the ministry Joni and Friends so those with disabilities will know the gospel and have their needs met with practical resources.

What is God going to do through us amid our trials? How can those things that feel like death to us bring life to someone else? There is a time for everything, and this is the moment to consider how we can do the good works God has prepared for us. We cannot wait until we are healed or until life seems easier to begin fulfilling our callings. May we be so abandoned to Jesus that even our most gut-wrenching losses become ministries of life and peace because He is in the midst of them.

Pray: Dear God, there are times when I am inspired by those who have conquered adversity. But sometimes I am discouraged when I compare their inspirational stories with my own life. Thank You for using their lives to ignite hope and bring comfort. Please forgive me for comparing my calling with theirs. Teach me how to use the comfort You give me to comfort others. In Jesus's name, amen.

Embrace: My most gut-wrenching losses can become ministries of life and peace when Jesus is in the midst of them.

Practice: What would people learn if they read a book about your life? Your story is still being written—is there anything you need to change in order to turn your life story into a tale of greater faith, persistence, and hope? Write down one thing that you would like to change. Pray daily for God to give you wisdom and help you take action steps to make that change possible.

Worship: "I Speak Jesus" by Charity Gayle, featuring Steven Musso

It's Never Too Late

Because of the LORD's great love we are not consumed, for his compassions never fail. They are new every morning; great is your faithfulness.

—*Lamentations 3:22–23*

Do you struggle to find reasons to be grateful when you are not feeling well? A number of years ago, during a season of worsening health, I prayed for God to help me teach gratitude to my teenage children. The Lord gently spoke to my spirit and said, *You will teach them by being grateful. Be an example to them.* God answered my prayer by convicting me in the area of one of my deepest struggles. My failure to cultivate gratitude in the midst of debilitating pain had affected my children's earlier years, but I was believing the lie that it was too late for me to change. That day, I embraced the truth that it is never too late for God to change someone.

Have you allowed illness and pain to produce an ungrateful heart within you? Have you, like me, made excuses for being ungrateful or discontented? Maybe you're thinking, *I am too old to change.* But advanced age never justifies sin. Or maybe your excuse is *Nobody knows the trauma I have endured.* Jesus knows; He will guide you toward healing and wholeness when you walk with Him.

It is never too late to nurture a grateful heart. The exercise of praise strengthens gratitude. The discipline of giving thanks teaches you to notice God's provision in your life. Are you ready to embrace your blessings instead of bemoaning your struggles? Let gratitude show you the way.

Pray: Dear God, forgive me for bemoaning my difficulties instead of recounting Your faithfulness. Help me develop a thankful spirit. Remind me that gratitude strengthens my faith. Thank You that it is not too late to practice the discipline of thanksgiving. Your mercies are new every morning. Today I will be grateful. Amen.

Embrace: It is never too late for me to nurture a grateful heart.

Practice: We all struggle with a discontented or ungrateful heart. Have you tried thanksgiving as a cure? Begin giving thanks to God for five things every day, and build your practice from there.

Worship: "Praise on the Inside" by J. Moss

You Still Have Something to Offer

—————|———————|—————

God's gifts and his call can never be withdrawn.
—*Romans 11:29, NLT*

G od gives divinely empowered abilities, or gifts, to every believer for the purpose of building up the body of Christ. Your illness cannot take away the gifts God gave you, but it can change the way they operate in your life. My gifts of teaching and encouraging are best used in relationship with others, so becoming mostly home-bound meant I had to get creative in searching for new ways to exercise those gifts. Like Paul, I decided that "if I am to go on living in the body, this will mean fruitful labor for me" (Philippians 1:22). It is not lost on me that Paul wrote this while he was in chains. Although the chains of illness may bind us, we are still free to use our God-given gifts.

Has illness limited *your* physical capabilities or ability to work? You might be discouraged. You may believe that there is nothing that you can contribute. But you still have gifts that illness cannot take away. Ask God how you can best use them during this season of life. Can you pray for someone? Perhaps you can speak a word of encouragement to a caregiver or helper today. You might even look for ways you can give to others who are ill. There may be something you can do that you have not yet considered. You still have something to contribute, so don't let your illness keep you isolated. Look for ways you can use your gifts to bless others. It is the Lord Christ you are serving, and you will be rewarded for your work.[4]

Pray: Dear God, thank You that illness does not change Your calling on my life. You knew the health struggles I would face, and You gave me gifts I can still use to bless others. Please keep me from being stuck in the past or thinking that I must be healthy before using my gifts. Open my eyes to the ways I can continue to serve You and bless others. Develop the gifts You have given me, even the ones I may not have discovered yet. In Jesus's name, amen.

Embrace: My illness cannot take away the gifts God gave me, but it can change the way they operate in my life.

Ponder: What are your spiritual gifts? If you do not know, ask your church for resources. There are also websites that offer free tests to help you discover the gifts God has given you. Take a moment to pray that He would show you how you can still use your gifts during this season of illness.

Worship: "The Cause of Christ" by Kari Jobe

A Healthy Appetite

Solid food is for the [spiritually] mature, whose senses are trained by practice to distinguish between what is morally good and what is evil.

—*Hebrews 5:14*, AMP

After I became sick, I consumed anything that might promote wellness. I took the medications the doctors prescribed. I sought out natural means of healing and began taking vitamins and supplements. I even avoided foods that cause inflammation and started eating healthier foods. For many years, I have not eaten gluten, dairy, red meat, or anything that has sugar. At first it was not easy, because I have an almost insatiable sweet tooth. But after a few months, I noticed that I did not crave chocolate or candy. Instead, I began to develop a voracious appetite for leafy greens, carrots, oranges, and blueberries. Now we can hardly keep enough fruits and veggies in the house! It turns out that avoiding junk food has given me a greater hunger for the things that nourish me.

Do you want to grow a stronger faith that can withstand the difficult trials that come with illness? You must nourish your spirit if you are to grow your faith. Stop chewing on bitterness, anger, gossip, or any other sins that are like poison food for your soul. Refuse to keep ordering from sin's harmful menu, and instead, develop increasing hunger for the things that are best for your spirit. God's Word is spiritual food that builds a strong spirit, but when you read Scripture without putting it into practice, you have just chewed up the finest meal but spit it out again. You will never nourish, or bring life to, your spirit that way. Being obedient to God's Word is how you digest truth so it can build strong faith.

Pray: Dear God, please help me nourish my spirit so I can withstand the difficulties that come with illness and affliction. Teach me how to follow You. Show me any hidden sin that hampers my walk with You. Forgive my transgressions. Give me a hunger for Your Word, and help me put it into practice. Help me grow up in my faith so I will be ready to receive solid food that satisfies. In Jesus's name, amen.

Embrace: Being obedient to God's Word is how I digest truth so it can build strong faith.

Practice: In what ways has obedience to God's Word built your faith? Ask Him to reveal any hidden sin that hinders your growth. Then read and pray the words of Psalm 51:9–12.

Worship: "Create in Me a Clean Heart" by Rusty Nelson and Integrity's Hosanna! Music

The Hospital Gift Shop

Joshua set up at Gilgal the twelve stones they had taken out of the Jordan. He said to the Israelites, "In the future when your descendants ask their parents, 'What do these stones mean?' tell them, 'Israel crossed the Jordan on dry ground.'"
—*Joshua 4:20–22*

It was spring, and I had just learned that I needed to endure yet another difficult surgery. Upon leaving my doctor's office, I noticed a beautiful Easter display in the hospital-gift-shop window. It featured the usual Easter eggs and stuffed bunnies, but there were also multiple shelves full of decorative crosses. I bought a ceramic cross as a proclamation of faith that God would help me through the surgery and its aftermath. He helped me, but it was not easy. My doctor made a life-threatening medical error. Thankfully, we discovered the reason behind my complications before it was too late. And five weeks after my initial surgery, I was back in the hospital for an emergency appendectomy. That season of surgeries and complications seemed like it would go on forever. But it didn't. The gift-shop cross now sits on my fireplace mantel. It serves as a visual reminder that difficult times have an expiration date but God's faithfulness is forever.

Pray: Dear God, thank You for all You have helped me through and all You *will* help me through. Help me establish visual reminders of Your faithfulness during difficulties. May my heart overflow with gratitude when I see them and remember Your goodness to me. My current health challenges can seem overwhelming until I recall all the ways You have met my needs in the past. Like the Israelites, I want to tell other generations about the amazing things You have done in my life. Amen.

Embrace: Difficult times have an expiration date, but God's faithfulness is forever.

Practice: Do you have anything that reminds you of a specific way that God has helped you in the past? Have you shared your story with anyone? It is not enough to simply remember when we look at our rocks of remembrance. Let us share our memories to help build the faith of those around us.

Worship: "We Will Remember" by Tommy Walker

Tucked Within His Love

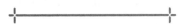

He will cover you with his feathers, and under his wings you
will find refuge; his faithfulness will be your shield and rampart.
—*Psalm 91:4*

The windows in the front of my house offer a vantage point
from which I can watch our Bradford pear tree as it grows and
changes with each new season. Today is a blustery day in November,
and an abundance of leaves are waving around in the wind and
shouting a last hurrah before they fall. I had just commented to my
children that I don't like the way our tree looks so shapeless and un-
tamed. However, as I watched it being buffeted about this morning,
I saw a bird making its way out of the tree's depths. The multitude of
leaves was protecting that little creature from the increasing cold and
winds of fall in Texas.

This scene reminded me of a story I heard years ago. There was an
art contest during the Vietnam War, and artists were supposed to
depict their interpretation of the word *peace*. The contestants entered
many creative pieces, but the winner had a rather unusual interpretation. His painting showed a bird's nest in a tree that was being rav-
aged by a roaring waterfall. In the middle of the nest was a bird
sheltering her young under her wing. This was peace. Peace wasn't
depicted as the absence of turmoil—it was the presence of a safe place
in the midst of it.

A cyclone of increased pain, new diagnoses, and concerns about
medical bills is whirling through my life. I desperately need a place of
peace. First I build my nest out of the promises in God's Word. Then
I take shelter under God's wing of protection. He becomes my refuge.

I am tucked within the comfort of His love while the storm still rages around me. I am no longer frightened, so I open my eyes. He is so close to me that now He is all I can see. Let it rain. I have found a place of peace in this storm.

Pray: I need You, God. You are my everything. I cannot and will not sit this storm out alone. I will not let it toss me about like a bird flying against the wind. It is fruitless and exhausting to fight against these trials by myself. When I am in the depths of sorrow, help me nest in Your truth. Give me faith that looks up to see Your outstretched wing. You will never leave me or forsake me. You are my peace. I love You. In Jesus's name, amen.

Embrace: I can find peace amid the storm when I am tucked within the comfort of God's love.

Practice: Read Galatians 5:22–25. Peace is a fruit of the Spirit. Do you need to rid yourself of anything that hampers the growth of this fruit in your life? How will you live by the Spirit today?

Worship: "Perfect Peace" by Laura Story

Rely on Your Helper

Do not quench [subdue, or be unresponsive to the working and guidance of] the [Holy] Spirit.
—1 Thessalonians 5:19, AMP

Imagine what it was like for faith-filled people who lived before Jesus gave the gift of the Holy Spirit. They had to live without the indwelling Holy Spirit to guide and strengthen them. Today as believers, we may have physical pain and illness, but we also have something that far outweighs any suffering: the Spirit of God, who lives in us. It may seem contradictory to have weak flesh and powerful Spirit residing together, but the Lord says, "My grace is sufficient for you, for my power is made perfect in weakness" (2 Corinthians 12:9). This grace and this power, available through the Holy Spirit, are given to all believers in Jesus Christ.

Severe health challenges exhaust our human ability to produce joy, but the Holy Spirit is a source of unending joy. Declining health causes our strength to fail, but the Holy Spirit strengthens us so we can endure any health challenge. The Holy Spirit is our helper. He even helps us guard against the temptations common to those who live with pain. Loneliness and pain often lead to excessive online shopping, unhealthy social media use, or even substance abuse. Being filled with the Spirit gives us the wisdom and self-control necessary to prevent us from overfilling ourselves with activities or substances that numb the mind as well as the pain. We must fully rely on the Spirit, who never fails, instead of depending on the flesh that has already failed us. Whether you are healthy or not, the Holy Spirit equips you to continue the calling that the Lord has given you. God has not abandoned you during illness. He has given you an eternally powerful helper.

Pray: Thank You, God, that I do not have to experience illness without the indwelling power of Your Holy Spirit. Thank You for giving me abundant life so even though I may be outwardly wasting away, You inwardly renew me to make me whole. Help me be filled with the Holy Spirit instead of being weighed down by sin that quenches the Spirit. Give me greater sensitivity to the many ways that Your Spirit works in my life. Thank You for the endurance and steadfast perseverance that You give me as I rely on You. Let me be a living testimony to Your power. In Jesus's name, amen.

Embrace: The indwelling power of the Holy Spirit helps, guides, and equips me to withstand the challenges of illness.

Ponder: The Bible teaches that God, Jesus, and the Holy Spirit are all one. How can dismissing the work of the Holy Spirit keep you from embracing all God wants for you? How can you stay sensitive to the work of the Spirit in your life?

Worship: "Spirit Lead Me (Live)" by Influence Music and Michael Ketterer

My Real Malignancy

Jesus spoke to them at once. "Don't be afraid," he said. "Take courage. I am here!"

—*Matthew 14:27, NLT*

Although my oncologist says my cancer seems to be growing at a "glacial" pace, it has quickly spread throughout my thoughts. It is a mental malignancy that, left unchecked, rapidly divides into discouragement, self-pity, and, finally, hopelessness. An arsenal of weapons, such as chemotherapy and biologics, are available to stop the spread of cancer. But what can fight my malignancy of thought? I can fight that only with weapons that "are not the weapons of the world. On the contrary, they have divine power to demolish strongholds" (2 Corinthians 10:4). How do we use weapons like those? The answer is in the next verse: "We demolish arguments and every pretension that sets itself up against the knowledge of God, and we take captive every thought to make it obedient to Christ" (verse 5).

Thoughts of fear, hopelessness, or despair about the future set themselves up against the knowledge of God. When I worry about needing more treatment for cancer or for any other illness, I am really predicting that my suffering will be too much to bear. Such speculations block out the reality of God's authority and presence in my life. Recognizing this brings freedom. I choose instead to take these malignant thoughts to God in prayer. When I confess my worries about the future and my fears of more suffering, He simply says, *I am here,* and I am comforted at last. So, yes, I still have cancer. But I also have a God who uses everything—even illness—to bring about His best for my life. And in this I rejoice.

Pray: Dear God, sometimes I fear facing a future that might be filled with more health issues. Stop me when I entertain fearful thoughts that predict a future without Your ample provision and strength. Forgive me for thoughts that deny the reality of Your omnipotence, omniscience, and omnipresence. Thank You that I can take courage because You are always here. You will never leave or forsake me. Help me rest in that knowledge today. In Jesus's name, amen.

Embrace: I will not allow fearful, discouraging, or hopeless thoughts to captivate me; I will take them captive to Christ.

Practice: How does recognizing God's sovereignty and faithfulness help you surrender your fears about the future? Write today's scripture on an index card, and place it near your bed. Give thanks for Jesus's constant presence in your life whenever you read it.

Worship: "My Weapon" by Natalie Grant

The Blessing of Contentment

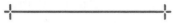

I have learned the secret of being content in any and every situation, whether well fed or hungry, whether living in plenty or in want. I can do all this through him who gives me strength.
—*Philippians 4:12–13*

It is a blessing to find contentment during illness. Contentment does not mean that we embrace illness; it means that we embrace God's strength to endure in the midst of it. But I have been reprimanded by well-meaning Christians who mistakenly believe that my peace and contentment during affliction are signs that I am not accepting God's best for my life. One friend actually said, "Don't you believe that God can heal you? Don't accept illness; it is not God's will for you to be sick and disabled!" Have you had people tell you this? What a burden it lays on those who are already suffering. I do not presume to know God's reason for allowing health issues in my life, but I trust that He is sovereign over all that concerns me.

The Great Physician is fully able to heal any ailment, and we might even experience the miracle of physical healing during this life. But if the miracle we so desperately desire is delayed until heaven, God will give us all we need to patiently endure the wait. Contentment and peace are just two of the beautiful ways God helps us persevere when we suffer from health challenges. He who overcame the world equips and enables us to overcome everything we face in this life. Overcoming illness sometimes looks like miraculous healing, but it can also look like miraculous strength, peace, and perseverance amid overwhelming suffering. Be encouraged. Jesus gives you all you need to triumph today and every day.

Pray: Dear God, I believe You can heal me today and will heal me for eternity. I long for complete restoration now, but I trust Your plan for my life even when I do not understand it. Grant me the contentment that comes from knowing that "I can do all things through Christ who strengthens me" (Philippians 4:13, NKJV). Fill me with Your Holy Spirit so I will have the power to persevere through any trial that tests my faith. Thank You for Your compassion and care for me. In Jesus's name, amen.

Embrace: The secret of contentment during health issues is that I can do all things through Jesus Christ, who gives me strength.

Ponder: How do you explain the difference between contentment and resignation regarding your health issues? Have you found contentment by trusting the Lord and relying on His strength during illness? Why or why not?

Worship: "Yet Not I but Through Christ in Me" by CityAlight

Keeping Healthy Days Healthy

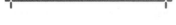

Wisdom is better than strength.
—*Ecclesiastes 9:16*

Do health issues ever prevent you from finishing a job or chore? Do you have any special hobbies or activities that you are unable to do on tougher days with illness or pain? We experience a growing pressure when illness prevents us from accomplishing things. The pressure propels us into excessive activity when a "healthy" day finally comes along.

Having a rare day when you are not overcome by health issues can be a heady experience. Newfound energy and strength make us bold enough to push ourselves. We might even ignore increasing pain and fatigue until it is too late. Have you ever done that? I have, and I always end up back in bed with an aching body that feels like it has been run over by a bus. Have you been there too? Then you need a plan for keeping "healthy" days healthy.

The solution is to plan ahead to pace yourself. Make a list of the things you can do on the days when you feel better. Prioritize them. When a good day comes along, try to complete one demanding item or two less-demanding items from your list. Then rest and reevaluate your ability to continue working. Your actions should be guided by wisdom and not by the strength you feel on your better days. Employing the wisdom to pace yourself may even help you experience a greater number of "healthy" days.

Pray: Dear God, thank You for the days when I feel better. Guide me with Your wisdom on my good days. Help me do the things that You have called me to do. Please teach me how to have a healthy balance so that I might have more good days. Grant me Your wisdom for when I am unable to do much at all. Help me not lose hope during those difficult times. I trust You with all my days because I belong to You. In Jesus's name, amen.

Embrace: My actions will be guided by wisdom and not by the strength I feel on my better days.

Practice: Does using up all your strength on a good day worsen your pain or fatigue the following days? Why is it important to plan the activities you want to accomplish on your better days? Begin making your list of them today!

Worship: "Wisdom Song" by Laura Woodley Osman

Asking for a Favor

✠──────────✠

"When did we see you sick or in prison and go to visit you?" The King will reply, "Truly I tell you, whatever you did for one of the least of these brothers and sisters of mine, you did for me."
—*Matthew 25:39–40*

Have you ever asked someone to help out a friend or family member as a favor to you? I was worried about my fourteen-year-old son during my hospitalization for cancer complications. He was home alone, and I wanted him to know I was thinking about him. My son and I loved to visit a smoothie shop near our house—it was our special thing to do together—so I reached out to a friend and asked her to surprise him with his favorite smoothie. I was bold enough to ask her because I love my son; my friend was happy to do something to help because she loves me.

Jesus taught that those who visit you or take care of you when you are sick are doing something for Him. Jesus is bold enough to ask others to visit us and care for us when we are sick, because He loves us. He never leaves us alone in our suffering, and He instructs others to come alongside to help us. Did you know that Jesus will reward those who faithfully obey Him? It is humbling to have people visit or take care of you. But there is eternal blessing in store for those who obey Jesus's admonition to help those who are sick. Caregiving is a God-given, sacred trust. Let us do all we can to ensure we do not make it difficult for others to help or visit us when we are sick.

Pray: Dear Jesus, thank You for telling Your followers that when they help those who are ill, they are helping You. Thank You for the people who help me and visit me. Bless them for their eagerness and willingness to be there for me. Help me accept their support and receive their help with a grateful heart instead of guilty shame for needing it. I will not stand in the way of their blessing. Amen.

Embrace: Caregiving is a God-given, sacred trust, so I will not make it difficult for others to help or visit me when I need care.

Ponder: Do you feel guilty when people visit you or take care of you when you are sick? How does it help you to know that Jesus asks His followers to do this work for Him?

Worship: "How He Loves" by David Crowder Band

Our Divemaster

Where can I go from your Spirit? Where can I flee from your presence? If I go up to the heavens, you are there; if I make my bed in the depths, you are there. . . . Even there your hand will guide me, your right hand will hold me fast.
—*Psalm 139:7–8, 10*

German theologian Julius Richter is credited with saying, "The burden of suffering seems to be a tombstone hung around our necks. Yet in reality, it is simply the weight necessary to hold the diver down while he is searching for pearls." Has the weight of suffering pulled you down into the watery depths of pain? You do not have to drown in despair; you have a divemaster who equips you with everything you need to navigate difficult waters. Jesus Christ already made the dive into suffering and death and victoriously resurfaced into the light of life. You can trust Him to safely lead you through an ocean of pain, because His loving care for you reaches into every depth.

A treasure diver can forget to use his diving equipment and be overcome by fear in the dark waters, or he can follow the divemaster's light, breathe one breath at a time, and begin searching for treasure. It may not seem like it right now, but God will use the full weight of your suffering to lead you to lasting treasures.

Pray: Dear God, You alone know the depths of my suffering. Use the weight of my pain to press me closer to You. Help me receive Your compassion for me. Take away my fear. Open my eyes so I may see the blessings You have given me during this time. Teach me how to breathe when I am in the depths. Bring light into my darkness, and illuminate the treasure You have for me today. Thank You that You will never leave me or forsake me. In Jesus's name, amen.

Embrace: God is using the full weight of my suffering to lead me to lasting treasures.

Ponder: A divemaster is in charge of an underwater-diving expedition. What qualities and experience would a divemaster need in order to lead others on a dive? How does Jesus perfectly fulfill the role of our divemaster?

Worship: "In Control" by Ke'Erron Sims, featuring Justin Cellum

Heartfelt Longings

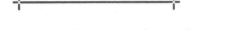

All my longings lie open before you, Lord; my sighing is not hidden from you.

—Psalm 38:9

After my first five years of living with chronic pain and illness, I wrote the following in my journal:

The Lord knows my longings. He knows that I desire to actively serve Him. During this very long season, it is hard to imagine that I am bringing glory to God as I lie here in bed. Yet I know that the Lord has chosen my path; He knows my longings. He sees the desires of my heart and promises to satisfy them as I trust in Him and delight in Him. I will trust Him to use everything, even my suffering and limitations, to fulfill the desires that He placed within me.

Chronic pain and illness change our lives dramatically. Those of us who live with debilitating health issues know that they affect our ability to pursue certain dreams. One of my dreams is to tour impressionist museums in France with my art-loving daughter, but I cannot endure a physically active trip right now. This dream may or may not come to fruition, but the heartfelt longing behind it is to build a beautiful relationship with my daughter. My dreams are simply specific ways that I want my longings to be fulfilled.

My dreams may change, but God gave me the heart's desire, or longing, to be a godly influence in my daughter's life. I trust Him to help me fulfill this longing, even if the path of fulfillment leads through the difficulties of being homebound instead of into art museums. What are some of your longings? You can trust God with them. He can satisfy the desires of your heart in ways you never dreamed were possible. Your creator understands your deepest longings. Surrender them to God; if they are part of His plan for you, not even illness can keep them from being fulfilled.

Pray: Dear God, Your Word tells me to delight myself in You and You will fulfill the desires of my heart. I delight in Your goodness. I delight in Your love. Illness has taken away so much that the road ahead of me can seem like a dead end, but You excel in making a way where there seems to be no way. You know the desires of my heart, and You know the things I would still love to accomplish. I submit my life, and all my desires, to Your care. Open my eyes to the ways You are already fulfilling my deepest longings. In Jesus's name, amen.

Embrace: When I find my delight in the Lord, He will satisfy the longings of my heart in ways that I never dreamed were possible.

Ponder: How does trusting and delighting in the Lord begin to reshape your heart's desires? Have your longings changed over time as your faith matures? How? What desire are you trusting the Lord with today?

Worship: "Jesus My Treasure" by Canyon Hills Worship

Becoming a Persistent Pray-er

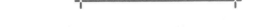

Jesus was telling the disciples a parable to make the point that at
all times they ought to pray and not give up and lose heart.
—*Luke 18:1*, AMP

Have you prayed for healing for yourself or others? Have you given up because you do not see any difference or because the illness seems to be getting worse? We often give in to discouragement when our prayers are not quickly answered in the way we had hoped. Do you ever quit praying about something when you do not receive an immediate answer? Persisting in prayer transforms us; God uses our prayer conversations to develop confident trust in Him. Continued and expectant prayer builds our relationship with God because we begin to depend on Him for everything.

Do not quit praying; your faith will grow as you begin seeing how God answers your prayers. The answers may not look like what you expected when you started to pray. Sometimes we receive more than we ask for; other times we must trust God's purpose and plan even when we do not understand it. Do you want to develop your faith? Keep praying. Do you want to know God better? Keep praying. Do not lose heart. Pray continually, expectantly, and with all persistence. Remember that persistent prayer builds faith that persists.

Pray: Dear God, I confess that I have often been quick to stop praying when I do not receive an immediate answer. Please forgive me. Thank You for telling me that You *want* me to persist in prayer. You desire to give me good gifts, but I must come to You in confident and expectant trust. Please transform my prayer life so that my faith in You will increase. In Jesus's name, amen.

Embrace: I will pray continually and expectantly; persistent prayer builds faith that persists.

Practice: Have you ever stopped praying about something when you did not get an immediate response? If so, does that issue still burden your heart? Write a letter to God, and pour out your feelings and hopes about your prayer request. Then pray about it!

Worship: "Because of Your Prayers (Grandma's Song)" by Anthony Evans

Straighten Your Thoughts

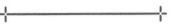

In your righteousness, rescue me and deliver me; turn your ear to me and save me.

—*Psalm 71:2*

One day about a decade ago, I woke up and immediately began to have discouraging, depressing, and ultimately life-robbing thoughts. I nursed them. I encouraged them. I started down a thought path toward hopelessness and despair, until I heard the Holy Spirit speak within me. His voice commanded me, *Straighten your thoughts!* It was bold. Powerful. Jarring. And it woke me from the world of lies in which I was dwelling.

Remember the scene in the movie *The Wizard of Oz* when Dorothy and her friends were being lulled to sleep in the field of poppies? One of them recognized that falling asleep would mean certain death and shouted a warning that awakened them. Like Dorothy, my mind was beginning to be numbed by something that could lead directly to the grave. Just as Dorothy's friend alerted her, my dearest friend and the Helper of my soul awakened me with truth to show me the way out.

Which thoughts need straightening in your own life? Begin to name them aloud and bring them into the light! Write them down. Tell them to Jesus. Then tell them to someone who can pray with you about them. And if you do not know which thoughts are straight and which are crooked (which way leads to life and which leads to death), talk to your pastor or a friend who knows and believes Scripture. Read the truth for yourself: Study the Bible to find verses that help you line up your thoughts with the truth that brings freedom. Write the verses on index cards. Place them next to your bed, on your mirror, and anywhere else that you might spend time. Leave them around your home as you would photos of loved ones. They are life and peace to you.

Pray: God, thank You that You are my helper. You lead me to triumph in Christ by teaching me wisdom's ways and guiding me on straight paths. You guard the paths of the just and protect those who are faithful to You, even when they go astray. Forgive me when I wander. Always lead me back to You, for You are my rescuer. Help me recognize when I am nurturing thoughts that do not lead to life. Give me the courage to speak to others about this so that I am not alone in my struggle. Thank You for loving me. In Jesus's name, amen.

Embrace: Scripture helps me line up my thoughts with the truth that brings life-giving freedom.

Practice: What kinds of thoughts do you nurture when you are sick or in pain? Have you noticed that your thoughts influence your feelings? Record what steps you will take to orient your thoughts toward life and peace.

Worship: "Need You Now (How Many Times)" by Plumb

Note: *Please get help if you are currently struggling with deep despair or thoughts of self-harm. See "Where to Find Help" on page 268 of this book. You are not alone; restore your hope by reaching out for help today.*

Generous Giving

Calling his disciples to him, Jesus said, "Truly I tell you, this poor widow has put more into the treasury than all the others. They all gave out of their wealth; but she, out of her poverty, put in everything—all she had to live on."

—*Mark 12:43–44*

Have you read the gospel account of the widow who gave a few cents to the temple treasury? She gave all she had without fanfare, but Jesus knew she had given all her money. Scripture does not tell us why her resources were limited, but her act of faithfulness demonstrated complete trust that God would take care of her. Biblical commentator Matthew Henry captured the idea of giving of oneself despite poverty, opposition, or suffering when he wrote that Jesus taught His disciples "to do what they can, when they cannot do what they would."[5] What a precious truth for those of us whose resources of energy or ability are limited by illness. We must do what we can when we cannot do what we would.

Have health issues taken away your resources? Perhaps they have limited your ability to provide for your family. Maybe afflictions have stolen your stamina. Jesus knew that the widow had given all she had to live on; He also knows the ways that illness has limited *your* resources. One of my daughters once said to me, "It's like the widow and the two coins. You do not have that much to give when it comes to physical stuff, but you give all you can." It is difficult to use up energy, strength, and stamina to give to others, particularly when it might cause pain. But "with God all things are possible" (Matthew 19:26). He is love; He opens up avenues for us to love and serve others despite our health issues. Sharing the riches of His love when you are experiencing the poverty of poor health brings a wealth of blessing.

Pray: Lord, bless my efforts to love others well. Like the woman who gave "all she had to live on" (Mark 12:44), show me how to be generous with my energy, strength, and time. May I never be so absorbed by my trials that I neglect your calling for my life. Please help me give generously even when my health is poor. Let illness be merely an avenue for Your glory to shine brightly. In Your name, amen.

Embrace: God will help me give generously of my energy, time, and strength even amid the poverty of poor health.

Practice: What are some ways you gave to others before you became ill? Have your health issues changed how you are able to minister to others? If you are grieving those losses, spend time in prayer and tell God how you feel. He cares for you.

Worship: "I Give Myself Away" by William McDowell

Tokens of Amazing Grace

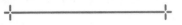

Rejoice in the Lord! It is no trouble for me to write the same things to you again, and it is a safeguard for you.
—*Philippians 3:1*

My floral teacup is filled with stories. This delicate cup holds some (now dried) pink roses that one of my children bought to celebrate my first year of remission from cancer. I recall that hard-won healing milestone whenever I look at it, but I remember something else when I look more closely: Nestled within the dried roses is a small wooden cross that I discovered in a parking lot five years before my cancer diagnosis. It tells a different story.

Hyperbaric oxygen therapy is considered an alternative treatment for CRPS, and it was my last-ditch attempt to regain the ability to walk without a walker. Although the procedures proved to be too expensive in Austin, my husband and I found a reasonably priced clinic in San Antonio. I spent the next six weeks living alone in a hotel near the clinic. I was desperate for healing, but I also desperately missed my husband and children. When I arrived at the clinic on the morning of my final treatment, I stepped out of the car and saw the wooden cross inscribed with the words "In Everything Give Thanks." I was already giving thanks! My CRPS pain was almost gone, and I could finally walk without my walker. The pressurized oxygen had worked powerfully on my limbs—that is, until four days later, when the crushing and burning pain returned with a vengeance. It is one thing to live every day with severe pain; it is entirely another to have it swoop in and clamp down after a period of freedom from it.

God knew I would need that wooden cross with those words, as the healing I'd hoped for did not come to pass. I learned to give thanks despite my heartache, pain, and tears. Purposefully thanking God during both crushing pain and shattering disappointment protected me from the dangers of despair. Determinedly rejoicing in the Lord is a valuable safeguard for my spirit.

Looks can be deceiving; inside my fragile floral teacup are two beautiful stories of strength. The cup holds the roses that celebrate my healing and commemorate the suffering I endured to be healed. The wooden cross celebrates the healing I will have one day, and it commemorates the suffering Jesus went through to make that possible. These tokens of God's amazing grace remind me that I have every reason to be thankful.

Pray: Dear God, thank You that Your strength lives within the fragile places of my life. You give me so many opportunities to discover Your provision; help me keep my spiritual eyes open so I will find it. Teach me to practice the discipline of rejoicing in You when my health issues threaten to engulf me. Thank You for every reminder of Your amazing grace. In Jesus's name, amen.

Embrace: Rejoicing in the Lord during every trouble and trial is a valuable safeguard for my spirit.

Ponder: Has your quest for healing led to disappointment? In what ways can rejoicing in God guard your spirit and faith during those challenges? What will you rejoice about and praise God for today? You can start right now!

Worship: "Hills and Valleys" by Tauren Wells

Every Step of the Way

The LORD says, "During the forty years that I led you through the wilderness, your clothes did not wear out, nor did the sandals on your feet."

—*Deuteronomy 29:5*

Almost every time I visit a doctor's office, they ask me to change into the gown or robe they provide. I have changed clothes for examinations, testing, and hospital stays. You have also likely changed into a robe for a short visit to the clean environment of a medical facility. So can you imagine traveling in a desert wilderness for forty years wearing the same clothes and shoes? This was the case for the Israelites before they entered the Promised Land, but God took care of them every single moment of those forty years. It is a miracle that their clothes and sandals did not wear out. My sandals seem to wear out after just a few summers in Texas, and I do not even walk very far! God provided His people with shoes and clothes that protected them every moment that they endured the rugged terrain. He has not changed; He will provide all that you need as you traverse the difficult landscape of illness. He will travel with you and care for you every step of the way.

Did you know that as He did with the Israelites, God has given us a covering for our feet? Our feet are covered with the peace that we have in Christ Jesus. The hope of our salvation will never wear out. Today we may endure the difficulties of the wilderness, but as the Israelites experienced before us, the Promised One walks with us on our way to the Promised Land. The depth and length of Christ's love help us walk through the depth of our pain and the length of our trials. His loving-kindness refreshes us during the heat of our hardship. He guides us through every difficulty. You will not travel through this landscape of pain and illness forever, but while you are here, God will provide for you every step of the way.

Pray: Dear God, You are faithful. Forgive me for the times when I am so focused on the landscape of my illness that I overlook the One who guides me through every difficulty. Open my eyes so I may see all the ways You provide for me: "When I said, 'My foot is slipping,' your unfailing love, LORD, supported me" (Psalm 94:18). Show me the wonder of Your great love. Transform difficult places into landmarks that show Your power. I love You. In Jesus's name, amen.

Embrace: The depth and length of Christ's love help me walk through the depth of my pain and the length of my trials.

Ponder: The Israelites wandered the desert for forty years with clothes and shoes that did not wear out. In what ways does that show God's loving concern for them? In what ways has God shown His love for you during your challenges and trials?

Worship: "He Knows My Name" by Master's Voice

Jesus Understands Suffering

———+———

I want to know Christ—yes, to know the power of his resurrection and participation in his sufferings, becoming like him in his
death, and so, somehow, attaining to the resurrection from the
dead. Not that I have already obtained all this, or have already
arrived at my goal, but I press on to take hold of that for which
Christ Jesus took hold of me.

—*Philippians 3:10–12*

I never understood what it meant to share in the suffering of
Jesus Christ until I experienced unrelenting chronic pain. The
lens of my misery sharpened my focus on the ways Jesus suffered for
us and with us. Do you have rebellious children? Jesus experienced
the heartbreak of parents longing to draw their wayward children to
themselves. Have you grieved the death of someone you love? Jesus
wept along with His beloved followers as they grieved a loved one's
death. Jesus also experienced the horrific loss of His cousin John,
and He responded by departing into "a solitary place" to pray (Mark
1:35).

Are you in a solitary place right now? Jesus has been there before
you. He most certainly understands your suffering. Let the depth of
your pain lead you to a greater love for the Savior, who chose to suffer for you. I have survived many years with deep, bone-crushing pain
because fellowship with Jesus gives me deep, despair-crushing comfort. Here is a portion of my journal from 2010, written after living
eight years with chronic pain:

On my worst pain days, I am alone in the peaceful and quiet comfort of my home. Jesus suffered a painful death before a mob of angry mocking people. I have my softest blankets, pillows, and clothing to ease my nerve pain; Jesus had a crown of thorns. I have cushioned orthotic shoes to protect my feet; Jesus had nails in His bare feet. I have medications and ointments to lessen my pain; Jesus had wine mixed with myrrh but refused to drink it. I have friends who comfort me and try to help with the burdens that are too much for me; all Jesus's friends ran away from Him in His time of need. One publicly disowned Him. Three times. Another friend was complicit in His murder. So, does He understand my pain and my sadness over the limits this disease places on me? Yes, all that and more. He is my comforter and companion. He does not condemn me or compare His wounds to mine; He merely lifts me out of the self-pity and loneliness of illness and encourages me to press on.

Pray: Dear God, thank You for choosing to suffer on my behalf. Forgive me for the times I have believed that You do not understand the depths of my suffering. Through Your Word, expose any other lies that keep me from receiving the fullness of Your comfort. Thank You that You are a compassionate God and extend that compassion to me. Help me experience the full measure of Your love today. In Jesus's name, amen.

Embrace: I can rejoice despite illness or deep, bone-crushing pain because fellowship with Jesus gives me deep, despair-crushing comfort.

Practice: Have you ever read the Gospels (Matthew, Mark, Luke, and John) in the New Testament, paying careful attention to the ways Jesus suffered? If not, why not start today?

Worship: "He Knows" by Jeremy Camp

Small Acts of Obedience

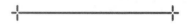

Work willingly at whatever you do, as though you were working for the Lord rather than for people. Remember that the Lord will give you an inheritance as your reward, and that the Master you are serving is Christ.
—*Colossians 3:23–24, NLT*

French theologian François de Salignac de La Mothe-Fénelon wrote,

Faithfulness ought not merely to lead us to do great things for His service, but whatever our hand finds to do, and which belongs to our state of life. The smallest things become great when God requires them of us; they are small only in themselves; they are always great when they are done for God.[6]

When illness is your constant companion, simply getting out of bed in the morning can require significant effort. The daily tasks that were done so easily, even joyfully, when you were healthy quickly become anxiety-producing burdens when you have health issues. Has illness turned small and formerly easy tasks into feats of enormous difficulty? Have those limitations led you to give up on your dreams of doing big things with your life? Perhaps it is time to examine how you measure your impact.

God's economy is different from ours. God uses the weak things of this world to shame the strong. He has chosen the poor to be rich in faith. He lifts up those who are bowed down. We may think that illness has kept us from doing big things for the Lord. But obedience to God in the things that may seem small, such as spending time in prayer or speaking an encouraging word, often brings the greatest gains. Instead of bemoaning all that illness prevents you from doing, faithfully attend to the small duties you can do each day. Ask God how you can bless others during this season of your life. Many small acts of obedience, strung together one after another, lead to a faith-filled life that has immeasurable impact.

Pray: Dear God, forgive me for using my limited understanding to measure the impact of my life. Please help me not to lean on my own understanding but to obey You in everything, even when I do not understand the reason. Help me complete the works You have prepared in advance for me to do. May my life be filled with eager expectation of Your goodness as I faithfully follow You. In Jesus's name, amen.

Embrace: Obedience to God in the things that may seem small often brings the greatest gains.

Ponder: Health issues may have forced you to quit doing important work or activities that brought great satisfaction to your life. How has your life changed because of your health issues? What is one "small thing" you can attend to every day?

Worship: "Yes (Obedience) (Live)" by David and Nicole Binion, featuring MDSN

My Quiet Times

> My heart is not proud, LORD, my eyes are not haughty; I do not concern myself with great matters or things too wonderful for me. But I have calmed and quieted myself, I am like a weaned child with its mother; like a weaned child I am content.
> —*Psalm 131:1–2*

Have you ever seen a newborn baby who is ready to be nursed? He will try to latch on to anything. An elbow. A chin. A pacifier. The harder an infant tries to get milk from something that does not produce it, the more frustrated he will become. I act just like that newborn when I neglect to spend quiet time with the Lord. Instead, I latch on to things that have no real power to nourish me and always end up frustrated.

Have you cultivated the habit of reading the Bible and praying every day? I usually spend time with God before I do anything else. For more than thirty years, my routine has been making my coffee and going to my floral rocking chair, where my Bible is waiting for me. I also have a journal, pen, and devotional nearby. First, I begin by asking God to teach me from His Word. Then I read my devotional and look up Scripture passages. I become immersed in the Bible, often losing track of time, before writing down the things God is teaching me.

But there are also days when I do not feel well enough to drink coffee or go to the room where I have my quiet times. On those days, it is crucial to make the choice to draw near to God, even if I never leave my bed. If I neglect the practice of seeking God first, I will quickly become weary and discontented because only He can satisfy my soul. Do you have days when spending time with God seems overwhelmingly difficult because of your illness? Do not neglect your quiet times; let the pressing needs of illness press you closer to the One who meets all your needs.

Pray: Dear God, forgive me when I fail to draw near to You. Thank you for the times when I feel better and become busy doing things I could not do when I was sick. Help me put You first on my better days. Sometimes I am overcome by pain, treatments, or side effects of medications. Help me put You first on my difficult days. Lord, I need you every day. Teach me to eagerly look forward to our times together. Call me into a deeper relationship with You. Instruct me from Your Word. Speak to me. Your servant is listening. In Jesus's name, amen.

Embrace: I am blessed that the God of the universe wants to spend time with me.

Ponder: Do you find it challenging to spend time with the Lord during tough seasons with illness? Why or why not? How can you soak in God's Word on difficult days? Perhaps you can listen to an audio Bible, such as Dwell, or watch a YouTube Scripture video series, such as Soakstream.

Worship: "Still" by Amanda Lindsey Cook

A Prescription for the Sick

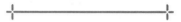

Is anyone among you sick? Let them call the elders of the church
to pray over them and anoint them with oil in the name of the
Lord.

—James 5:14

For years, I did not want to impose on the church elders to pray
for me during my debilitating illness. But then I was diagnosed
with aggressive cancer, and a serious surgical complication prevented
me from receiving chemotherapy. The cancer was rapidly growing
and spreading. Every moment counted. It was time to call the church
elders to pray.

Our pastor and a group of elders assembled in our home. They
anointed me with oil and prayed for healing. One man prayed over
the relentless lingering pain in my biopsy incision; it melted away
and never returned. God healed me in an instant, but my journey
toward cancer remission took longer. I do not know how He answered every prayer that day, but I do know that it was a miracle that
I lived through my cancer battle. A medical prescription sometimes
brings instant healing, but other times it gives you what you need in
order to manage and endure a difficult illness. Calling the elders to
pray for you is a biblical prescription for the sick.

Have you ever called your church and asked the elders to pray over
you? You may think your illness does not qualify for the attention of
your church elders. But the original Greek word for "sick" in James
5:14 is *asthenei*, and it means weak, feeble, and just plain sick! You do
not need to have a life-threatening illness to ask for prayer; you just
need humble obedience to call the elders to fulfill their divinely appointed ministry to pray for you.

Pray: Dear God, thank You for taking care of all my needs. Your Word is a guidebook for hardship in this life. Help me obey every part of it, including the admonition to call the elders to pray for me when I am sick. Thank You for our church leaders who work hard to serve You; bless them and their families. Protect them, and give them strength to serve You. Help them fulfill the roles You have established for them. Thank You for giving me a prescription for prayer when I am sick. In Jesus's name, amen.

Embrace: Prayer from church elders is a biblical prescription for those who are sick.

Ponder: Have you followed the biblical prescription to have your elders pray for you? Why or why not? If you do not currently attend church, go to "You Can Know Jesus" on page 261 for a website that can help you find a local Bible-believing church.

Worship: "Fighting for Us" by Anthony Evans

Observations from a Chronic-Pain Group

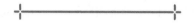

Don't look out only for your own interests, but take an interest in others, too.

—Philippians 2:4, NLT

When walking into my first chronic-pain support group, I looked around and thought, *These are my people.* But my hopes for a supportive meeting were dashed. Nearly every time someone shared their experience with chronic pain, other members immediately poured out their own similar—but worse—stories. There seemed to be a subtle, and at times not-so-subtle, competition to win the title of Worst Illness. The group members were so eager to be heard that they weren't listening to or regarding others.

One duo of unforgettable older ladies proved to be an exception. Their names are Trudy and Winnie. Trudy said that Winnie dragged her everywhere and she ended up exhausted and in bed for days. She finally had to tell her a firm no. Winnie just sat there beaming, unaffected. They were a hoot! The leader of our group said that these old buddies, who were both single, one because of the death of a spouse and the other because of divorce, were soulmates. These ladies were an example that God can provide the companionship you need at any stage of life.

One man in the group shared about his emotional struggles since he started living with debilitating pain. He questioned his purpose in life and confided that he was losing the will to live. Winnie immediately spoke up. She asked him, "What is one charity that you would love to help or do something for?"

He thought for a moment and finally suggested, "Homeless people."

Winnie was thrilled and shared, "I belong to a group called the Hippies."

This was Austin, Texas, after all.

She continued, "We don't sit around and drink or do drugs like you might think; we help the homeless!"

She invited this suffering man to join her in helping people. Winnie was so eager to give to others despite her own infirmities. She was truly a delight to behold.

Pray: God, I confess that there are times when I grumble and do not appreciate the abilities You have given me. Forgive my impatience with those who are so blinded by suffering that they cannot see anything else. I have also rushed to present my tale instead of first pausing to listen to people. Help me see past my own pain into the chasm of someone else's affliction. Let me not forget that friendships can grow from seeds of our related pain but blossom best when we work together to serve others. In Jesus's name, amen.

Embrace: Friendships can grow from seeds of our related pain but blossom best when we work together to serve others.

Practice: How does serving others help someone who is lost amid suffering to find purpose? Think of a friend who is struggling right now. Reach out, and brainstorm one way you can work together to bless someone. Have fun!

Worship: "Build My Life" by Pat Barrett

The Richest Soil

I will walk humbly all my years because of this anguish of my
soul. Lord, by such things people live; and my spirit finds life in
them too. You restored me to health and let me live. Surely it was
for my benefit that I suffered such anguish.
—*Isaiah 38:15–17*

I was a Christian for thirteen years before I became sick with chronic
pain. I loved being active in my church and at my job; I taught first
grade and later became a director of children's ministry. But my
greatest joy was being the stay-at-home mother of three children.
Life was busy and full. I was a homemaker who loved being a wife and
mom. Who had time for illness? Certainly not I!

Then I got an injection that triggered a severe autoimmune response. My pain grew worse and worse until it became difficult for
me to walk. I would lie in bed, muscles on fire, and tell my husband
that it felt like my body was dying. I was weak, in pain, and shocked
that the Lord had allowed this illness to take over my life. After all,
wasn't I a faithful servant? Hadn't I cultivated a close relationship
with God through daily prayer and Bible study? At that time, I did
not understand why He allowed me to experience such tremendous
suffering. But the truth is that I had conveniently skimmed over the
Bible verses that taught about affliction. Deep down, I believed my
faithfulness to God would protect me from pain. In my ignorance
and pride, I told Him that I did not need this degree of pruning to be
fruitful. But I did not even know what kind of fruit He was getting
ready to grow.

The Master Gardener knows what conditions are favorable for
seeds of humility and holiness to take root and grow. Before chronic

illness, I believed my heart was fully devoted to God. My suffering exposed areas of faithlessness and idolatry that I never knew existed within me. I was quick to judge, but I shielded my judgment under the umbrella of righteousness. Seeds of mercy and compassion cannot take root in that shade. God has grown a deeper love of mercy and given me compassion for others who suffer. The soil of my life has been made rich by adversity. The pretenses of self-reliance and pride are being destroyed, creating a rich fertilizer for the new seeds that God is planting within me. There will be a harvest. I just need to trust the Master Gardener. Surely it was for my benefit—and the benefit of others—that I suffered, and continue to suffer, such anguish.

Pray: Dear God, You know the depths of my pain and the challenge of adjusting to a life with health issues. I pray for complete healing. But until I am healed, please open my eyes to see the ways You allow illness to work in my life. Teach me to trust You. You are the Master Gardener; use my suffering to help me grow fruit that lasts. Thank You, God. In Jesus's name, amen.

Embrace: Adversity enriches the soil of my life so seeds of humility and holiness can take root and grow.

Ponder: Are you able to discern any benefits that have come out of your illness? Perhaps you have more compassion for others. Maybe you have deeper relationships and appreciate the small things in life. Pray that God would reveal one way that He is working through your illness, and then thank Him for it.

Worship: "The Garden" by Kari Jobe

Rocks in My Suitcase

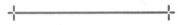

*You're going to wear yourself out—and the people, too. This job
is too heavy a burden for you to handle all by yourself.*
—*Exodus 18:18,* NLT

Our Bible study leaders offered to drive me to Houston for my
MD Anderson Cancer Center appointment. When they walked
into my house, they were surprised that I had packed two large bags
for a two-night stay. While lifting the heavier bag, one of them joked
that I must have packed rocks in my suitcase. I was forced to admit
that I had included a compact coffee maker, essential equipment for
waking up and getting ready to navigate a large hospital. My love of
coffee, and my overpacking, became the source of much amusement
to our Bible study group. It is less amusing when you realize my reasons for packing so much. The pillows, blankets, supplements, inhal-
ers, pain patches, and other items that accompany illness must come
with me during my travels.

Has illness changed the way you travel? You may be homebound
but need a back pillow for the ride to your doctor's office. Perhaps
a need to be near a bathroom limits your activity or causes you to
request an aisle seat on an airplane. We become so accustomed to the
myriad adjustments we make to accommodate illness that it is unset-
tling to suddenly view ourselves through another person's eyes.
When a healthy friend was helping me pack for a trip, she was surprised to learn that all my clothing was hung inside out. Since I am
typically fastidious, she asked, "Why do you hang clothes that way?"
I had no idea how to answer until I did laundry later that week. I realized that I did not turn my clothing right side out because the pro-

cess of placing the clothes on hangers made my hands hurt. I was subconsciously limiting my movements to prevent further pain. The realization made me feel sad.

How many ways do you accommodate illness, guard against pain, and attempt to prevent further complications? You are fighting a daily battle; no wonder you are fatigued! You may be dismayed when you begin to notice the ways that illness has changed how you function in the world. But there is beautiful freedom when you acknowledge and grieve the invisible load that illness causes you to carry. No, you are not putting rocks in your suitcases; you are carrying a heavy load. Give yourself permission to be sad about it.

Pray: Dear God, there are times when I almost forget my health issues. But there are days when I cannot help but notice the heavy burdens that illness compels me to carry. I am sad that illness has changed my life. Help me find creative ways to accommodate my health challenges. Teach me how to live well despite them. Bring people into my life who can help me carry this heavy load; help us lift our burdens to You. In Jesus's name, amen.

Embrace: There is freedom in acknowledging and grieving the invisible load that illness causes me to carry.

Ponder: God often sends people to help us when burdens are too heavy to handle by ourselves. What are some ways that others have helped you carry the burdens of illness? Thank them for how they have helped you.

Worship: "Joy Comes in the Morning (Live)" by Church of the City, featuring Tasha Layton

The Best Training Program

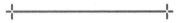

Physical training is of some value, but godliness (spiritual training) is of value in everything and in every way, since it holds promise for the present life and for the life to come.
—*1 Timothy 4:8, AMP*

I did not grow up in an athletic family, so it wasn't until I was almost out of high school that I discovered my love for exercise. It began with aerobics (this was the 1980s, after all), leading to a job teaching classes and training people on weight machines. Then I graduated and began taking summer classes at Auburn University, where I discovered my love for running. I ran during those brutally hot Alabama summer days. I ran during those balmy nights. People began to notice that I ran all the time, and a few of them asked me if I was in training. I was a little unsure what the term *in training* meant since I had never been an athlete, but I nodded my head. Then they asked, "What are you training for?" I was embarrassed by the looks I got when I said, "I'm training to be in good shape!" Apparently, being in training means different things to different people. I may not have been in training for a race or to be on a team, but every course of action to which we commit ourselves trains us for something.

Have you ever followed a prescribed training program? Perhaps you pursue good health by disciplining yourself to follow a recommended exercise, physical therapy, or nutritional plan. Better health is a terrific goal, but are you so fixated on having a healthy body that you neglect to pursue things that bring health to your spirit? What changes can you make to implement the same diligent training in your spiritual life? Reading the Bible, praying daily, and spending time in fellowship with others are spiritual exercises that will strengthen your faith. Loving others and finding ways to serve will help you develop your spiritual muscles so you will be strong in the Lord. Consider the ways you can train to endure the race ahead of you. Train your mind to dwell on praiseworthy things, train yourself to submit to Christ, and train your heart to love God and others. We are to "run in such a way as to get the [eternal] prize" (1 Corinthians 9:24), so train yourself to run toward the things that will last.

Pray: Lord, give me determination and diligence to follow the spiritual training You have prescribed for me. This course has been so challenging. Thank You that my challenges enable me to be a stronger runner. Help me use all the spiritual exercises available to me: obedience, submission, prayer, Bible study, fellowship, and service. Thank You for training and equipping me to persevere through everything that You have appointed for me. In Your name, amen.

Embrace: I will follow a disciplined spiritual-exercise program so I can persevere through this difficult race.

Ponder: It is easy to follow a diet or exercise program when we see quick results, and less so when the results come more slowly. The same is true in our spiritual lives: Sometimes we do not see immediate results from our efforts. Why is it crucial to continue building rhythms such as prayer and Bible study into our lives? What are some ways you can ensure that you persevere, even on the days when you want to give up?

Worship: "I'll Keep Running to You" by Todd Dulaney

Essential Ingredients

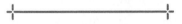

[With joy] let us exult in our sufferings and rejoice in our hardships, knowing that hardship (distress, pressure, trouble) produces patient endurance; and endurance, proven character (spiritual maturity); and proven character, hope and confident assurance [of eternal salvation].

—Romans 5:3–4, AMP

Have you ever watched the television show *Chopped*? Chefs compete with one another by making meals from ingredients in a mystery basket. Each basket contains unusual flavor combinations, which typically include anything from pigs' feet and candy to sardines and fruit. The combination of ingredients seems both random and unappealing, but a culinary team works behind the scenes to carefully craft each basket. Even the most unappetizing flavor combinations have been strategically chosen with the goal of a successful meal in mind. Competitors must solve the ingredient puzzle if they are to create the intended meal. The chefs receive additional ingredients and the tools they need to be successful, and the winner takes home a prize.

Have your health issues or hardships seemed as arbitrary and bewildering as the mystery-basket ingredients on *Chopped*? Mine certainly have! The trials you face may not seem related; they may appear as ill-conceived as the ingredients in those baskets. But your hardships have a common theme that you might discover if you look closely enough. What is the theme of your trials? It could be self-denial. Perhaps it's humility. The overarching purpose of hardship is no mystery—the purpose is always sanctification. God's masterful and loving intention for you is that your difficulties would help transform your life into one that brings glory to Him and unimaginable eternal reward to you.

The contestants on *Chopped* receive everything they need to successfully turn unappetizing ingredients into culinary masterpieces. God provides all that *you* need too! Trials and hardships produce spiritual maturity when you use the tools available to you. A joyful spirit, a thankful heart, and patient perseverance are just some of the equipment that will sweeten the bitterness and make something beautiful out of your difficulties. Remember that "his divine power has given us everything we need for a godly life through our knowledge of him who called us by his own glory and goodness" (2 Peter 1:3). Your relationship with Jesus and the equipping power of the Holy Spirit are the essential ingredients that make a glorious masterpiece of your life.

Pray: Dear God, thank You for using even the most unappealing ingredients in my life to create something beautiful in me. Teach me to use all the tools You provide so I can produce a life that brings glory to You. You began a good work in me, and You will bring it to completion. Thank You that You love me enough to refine my faith and strengthen my character. Give me the faith to trust Your plan. In Jesus's name, amen.

Embrace: The overarching purpose of my trials is no mystery—the purpose is always sanctification.

Ponder: Have you experienced so many trials and hardships that they seem as random and bizarre as the ingredients in the *Chopped* baskets? How are these difficulties shaping your character? If you are not sure, ask God to reveal the answer to you.

Worship: "Blessings" by Laura Story

Nothing Can *Take* My Life

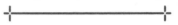

I give them eternal life, and they shall never perish; no one will
snatch them out of my hand.
—*John 10:28*

Two years after I completed chemotherapy, a CT scan showed that my non-Hodgkin lymphoma was advancing again. I needed a biopsy. My aggressive form of lymphoma was in remission, but I still had slow-growing lymphoma that my doctors consider to be incurable. I knew the cancer would continue to grow; however, I wanted anything but more cancer treatment. I wanted to travel. I wanted to experience the joy of having grandchildren. And I desperately wanted to finish writing my book of devotionals. But here it was again, the cancer that threatened my life and tried to rob me of the opportunity to fulfill my dreams.

The truth is, none of us can add or subtract an hour—or a minute or even a second—to or from our lives. In Psalm 139:16, David wrote that all the days God ordained for you were written in His book even before you were born! Illness cannot rob you of one moment of the life He has planned for you. God will fulfill His purpose for you, so you can trust that you will live until it is completed. Have you given your life to Jesus Christ? Then you belong to Him. Nothing can take away the eternal life He died to give you. If you trust the Lord with your eternal life, then how much more can you trust Him with the rest of your days on this earth?

Five years after my cancer relapsed, COVID invaded our world. Those of us with a difficult diagnosis or a complicated medical history had reason to be gravely concerned. Healthy concern must be anchored by both wisdom and truth so we will not drift into a sea of worries. Wisdom says, "Do not test the Lord. Use discernment while taking care of yourself and others." Truth says, "You do not belong to COVID, cancer, or any other disease. You belong to the Lord, and nothing can touch a hair on your head apart from the will of your Father in heaven. So do not fear." Nothing can ever *take* your life when you belong to Jesus.

Pray: Dear God, thank You for giving me the assurance and perspective of Your Word. The truth is that my spirit was dead before I accepted Jesus. My eternal life began when I accepted Him, and it will continue in heaven. Thank You that I do not need to fear death. Teach me to fully recognize the brevity of my days so I may live with wisdom. Help me complete the good works that You prepared for me, and give me great boldness in sharing the gospel so that others may live. In Jesus's mighty name, amen.

Embrace: All the days God ordained for me were written in His book even before I was born.

Practice: Jesus said, "I give them eternal life, and they shall never perish; no one will snatch them out of my hand" (John 10:28). How does this verse give peace to a believer with health issues? Write out this scripture or record it so you can commit it to memory.

Worship: "Promises" by Maverick City Music, featuring Joe L. Barnes and Naomi Raine

Pampering the Flesh

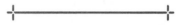

> You, my brothers and sisters, were called to be free. But do not use your freedom to indulge the flesh; rather, serve one another humbly in love.
>
> —*Galatians 5:13*

I seek out anything that gives me a bit of relief from pain and illness. I love comfortable clothes, soft beds, warm baths, and heating pads. But what I really love is when my pain quiets down and I feel like the old me: the person without any disease. My desire for comfort leads me to pamper myself with an endless array of products that promise to make my pain better. Perhaps my painful flesh will finally be satisfied and stop its reign of terror. But guess what? When you give in to terrorists' demands, they demand more—and so it is with the flesh. It is never fully satisfied, so I continue my endless journey to find the healing comfort my body craves.

Do you also depend on excessive comforts to endure your daily health battles? This can lead to a type of entitlement particular to those who live with chronic illness. We may begin to believe we deserve to have anything that brings us temporary comfort, whether it is truly good for us or not. Finding relief from the symptoms of illness can demand all our attention. Our friends may even give us permission for this growing self-absorption by saying, "Take care of yourself," then adding the statement that gives our innate selfishness carte blanche: "Just worry about *you* right now."

But do we want to think about only ourselves all the time? Chronic health issues can already cause isolation. Severe illness necessitates much discussion about our physical health, medications, and treatment, and life becomes deeply wearisome when we constantly focus all our attention on ourselves. We were designed for more. Our creator designed us to be in relationship with other people. Things may provide temporary comfort, but only God and the love of others can truly comfort us.

If your struggles with health issues have led to entitlement or selfish behavior, know that you have a Savior who has compassion for you. He is eager to forgive you and help you consider the needs of others. Illness does not exempt you from living the life of love that Scripture calls you to. It turns out that loving God and others can give you the soothing comfort that nothing else can ever provide.

Pray: Dear God, I know that I have often focused all my attention on my comfort. Forgive me. Please help me live for You instead of for ways to feel better. Teach me how to have a balance between taking care of myself and caring for others. You gave up every comfort when You came to earth to endure the cross for my sake; help me follow Your loving example. I am weak, but Your Holy Spirit lives in me; please strengthen me by Your Spirit. In Jesus's name I pray. Amen.

Embrace: Loving God and others gives me the soothing comfort that nothing else can ever provide.

Ponder: God's Word teaches us how to live lives of love and consideration for others; illness does not exempt us from this calling. Have you ever used your condition to excuse selfishness, impatience, or entitlement? Ask forgiveness from anyone you may have hurt by these behaviors.

Worship: "Less Like Me" by Zach Williams

Carrying a Heavy Cross

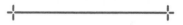

Whoever does not take up their cross and follow me is not worthy of me.

—*Matthew 10:38*

Illness has taught me how very much I crave comfort. I want to feel good at almost any cost. I will pay more for sheets that do not exacerbate nerve pain. I feel entitled to sit in the softest chair so my back will not hurt. And I rationalize my driving too fast with the thought that I absolutely need to get home and lie down. Yes, I certainly crave comfort. So how do I reconcile my attempts to function well with illness with Jesus's command to deny myself, take up my cross, and follow Him?

First I ask for help from the Lord by praying, "Today I feel as though the weight of this cross of illness has pinned me to the ground. I'd like to be free of it so I can more easily follow You, Jesus, but that is not Your design. Your design is that I take it up, carry it, and follow You. Help me do this, Lord, for I am so weak. May Your strength enable me to take it up and carry it. When I need help, send someone to help me carry this weighty thing so I may follow wherever You lead."

Jesus taught us how to follow Him when He said to His disciples, "Whoever wants to be my disciple must deny themselves and take up their cross and follow me" (Mark 8:34). When He spoke these words, the cross was not the decorative ornament it has become in our culture; rather, it was a fearsome and shameful instrument of public torture and death, and His disciples surely knew it. Yet Jesus instructed that whoever wants to be His follower must take up their cross.

If the cross is an instrument that puts the flesh to death, then what is *your* cross? If illness, pain, and suffering help you die to your worldly desires, they are indeed your cross. However, if you use suffering to excuse increasing overindulgence and self-absorption, it is merely a decorative cross with no eternal value. We carry the burdens of illness and pain either way. We can either pick them up and carry them to Jesus or wear them as a heavy weight that presses us more closely to this world. Today let us choose to pick up our cross, whatever it may be, and wholeheartedly follow Him.

Pray: Lord, help me deny myself today. Teach me how to live with illness so that it becomes an eternally valuable tool of transformation. Help me submit my entire life to You today. Give me the strength to take up the burdens that You have allowed for me. Teach me to follow Your servant-hearted ways. In Your name, amen.

Embrace: The cross I bear has a purpose: It is an eternally valuable tool of transformation in my life.

Ponder: What is your cross? Are you being pinned by the weight of it, or are you carrying it and following Jesus? Is anyone in the body of Christ helping you carry it?

Worship: "More Like Jesus (Live)" by Passion, featuring Kristian Stanfill

God of Miracles

Jesus Christ is the same yesterday and today and forever.
—*Hebrews 13:8*

Being diagnosed with debilitating health issues has changed how I read the Bible. Now I eagerly try to absorb every detail about the healing miracles Jesus performed. He lived among those who were hurting and who desperately needed a healer. They needed Jesus to perform miracles so they could believe God sent Him. The miracles that restored bodies and minds pointed those people toward faith that could save them. Faith in Jesus released them from the bondage of sin, which leads to eternal death; rather than just physical healing, they were given the miraculous gift of eternal life. So much was restored by His healing touch. The same is true for us today. So much is still restored by His healing touch.

I used to secretly wish that I had lived during Jesus's earthly ministry so I could receive healing, but my faith falters when I believe that His miracles were confined to a time that is long past. He is still alive, and He is still in the healing business. My single-minded pursuit of physical healing can cloud my mind and block my view of the ways that Jesus has already healed me. The truth is that I have already experienced healing miracles. My greatest healing happened spiritually when I accepted Jesus into my life. He healed me from the sting of sin and the curse of eternal death. My most remarkable *physical* healing happened when a receptionist at a surgical center told me that I could not take over-the-counter pain medication before my surgery. Then she laid her hand on my arm, and even before she opened her mouth to say, "God bless you," the intense burning pain instantly vanished.

The miracles have never ceased. Isn't it also a miracle to suffer daily from severe pain yet patiently and faithfully endure? My complete healing would be a powerful testimony. But perhaps God is choosing to display His power in a different way. I am a living example of the miraculous sufficiency of Jesus Christ; He gives me the strength and endurance to thrive while living with disabling pain and illness. Truly, He is still the God of miracles.

Pray: Dear Jesus, thank You that You never change. You still love us, and You still heal us. Open my eyes to the ways You are performing healing miracles in my life. Forgive me when I forget the ways You have already healed me. You healed my broken spirit by giving me a new spirit. You restored my relationship with God. You hold all my healing in Your hands. I will experience complete healing in Your timing. Grant me patience and endurance until that day. Amen.

Embrace: My single-minded pursuit of physical healing can cloud my mind and block my view of the ways that Jesus has already healed me.

Ponder: Do you trust that God has authority to heal but also has a purpose in your suffering that you might not understand? Why or why not? What is one way that you have already experienced His miraculous healing (spiritual, emotional, or physical)?

Worship: "Miracles (Live)" by Jesus Culture, featuring Chris Quilala

God Still Cares About You

"Because he loves me," says the LORD, "I will rescue him; I will protect him, for he acknowledges my name."
—*Psalm 91:14*

Illness can make us feel miserable, and our misery is compounded when we believe that no one cares about our suffering. Do you trust that God cares about you even during sleepless nights or pain-filled days? Or do you assume that He is not listening when your prayers for healing seem to go unanswered? Suffering will distort your perception of God unless you are firmly grounded in biblical truth. When you begin to lose faith in His loving character, an insidious pattern can appear in your spiritual life. Before long, you might decide that you are "too busy" for Bible study. You may even be tempted to give up on prayer. Have you ever noticed this shift in your life? Be assured that God has not ignored your suffering. He is always concerned about what concerns you.

We do not have to read far in the Bible to find an example of God's concern for human suffering. In Exodus, the second book of the Old Testament, we read that the Israelites were enslaved and oppressed in Egypt. In their misery, they began to cry out to God. What was His response to their prayers? "God saw the Israelites, and He took notice" (2:25, HCSB). The Hebrew word for "notice" in this verse is *yada,* and it implies deep knowledge coupled with action. God took action! He told Moses, "I have indeed seen the misery of my people in Egypt. . . . I am concerned about their suffering. So I have come down to rescue them" (3:7–8).

God excels at rescue operations. He rescued the Israelites from slavery through Moses. He rescues us from slavery to sin and death through Jesus. The God who hears prayers and takes action has not changed! He is concerned about you. He has seen your misery. How will you respond to His concern for you? The author of Exodus revealed that when the Israelites "heard that the LORD was concerned about them and had seen their misery, they bowed down and worshiped" (4:31). They were still enslaved, but they responded to God's care for them by bowing and worshiping. We do not have to wait for freedom from our health issues to worship the God who loves us.

Pray: Dear Lord, I worship You today. You are my savior and redeemer. You are worthy of my praise. Thank You for being concerned about me. Forgive me for the times when I doubt Your love for me. When I feel the isolation or misery of illness, remind me that You see me and care for me. When I feel oppressed by pain, remind me that You are my strength and my deliverer. Increase my faith and restore my soul so I will be steadfast. In Your precious name I pray. Amen.

Embrace: I will not wait for freedom from my health issues to worship the God who loves me.

Ponder: Does your suffering have the power to change God's character? Why or why not? What are three attributes of His character for which you are grateful today?

Worship: "Defender" by Francesca Battistelli, featuring Steffany Gretzinger

My Doctor Is Not My Savior

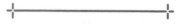

I, even I, am the LORD, and apart from me there is no savior.
—*Isaiah 43:11*

K ing Asa was severely ill, but he did not seek the Lord when he was stricken by illness. The author of 2 Chronicles explained,

In the thirty-ninth year of his reign Asa developed a disease in his feet. His disease was severe, yet even in his illness he did not seek the LORD, but [relied only on] the physicians. So Asa slept with his fathers [in death], dying in the forty-first year of his reign. (16:12–13, AMP)

Is it possible that Asa allowed his fear of disease to become greater than his fear of God? Sometimes people blame God when they become ill. They are angry that He allows their pain and suffering, so they follow Asa's example and seek only the advice of their physicians. But it is unwise to stop acknowledging the Lord in any area of your life. Notice what happened to Asa: He died two years later. His doctors could not save him, and they certainly could not save his soul. Only the Savior has the power to save us.

After a new diagnosis, do you seek answers from doctors, the internet, books, and any other source you can get your hands on? God has given us many ways to find the medical help we need, but we operate in a spirit of fear when we desperately search for worldly solutions and neglect to seek His wisdom. Sometimes He uses the skills of a wonderful doctor to heal us, but we cannot place the entirety of our hopes for healing in the hands of another human. When we do this, we are exalting them to a place that only God can occupy.

Doctors are tremendous sources of help; their medical training and commitment to healing can alleviate suffering and extend lives. But the God who created you knows every single cell of your body, so do not forget to seek His wisdom to guide your decisions during your health struggles. I am trusting creation above the Creator when I trust the hands of my medical team more than the God who created those hands. Let your eagerness for healing lead you to eagerly seek the Healer.

Pray: Dear God, thank You for providing the knowledge, compassion, and care of good doctors. They are a tremendous blessing, but only You are perfect. Please forgive me if I have expected perfection from my doctors. Help me remember that You alone are my creator, sustainer, and healer. You are the Savior who has given me eternal life. Forgive me if I have acted like King Asa and stopped relying on You. Restore a right spirit within me. Give me wisdom, and lead me toward greater health and healing. In Jesus's name, amen.

Embrace: Only the Savior has complete power to save me.

Practice: Have you prayed for your doctors, nurses, and care team? Pray for them right now. Ask God to give them wisdom as they care for patients. Pray that He will provide them with restoration and renewed spirits after difficult cases.

Worship: "Healer" by Casting Crowns

A Branding of Sufficient Grace

He said to me, "My grace is sufficient for you, for my power is made perfect in weakness." Therefore I will boast all the more gladly about my weaknesses, so that Christ's power may rest on me.

—2 Corinthians 12:9

The above Scripture passage inspired this entry in one of my old journals:

Sometimes God's servants are called to undergo suffering so severe it seems to brand their lives with pain. Paul's well-known thorn in the flesh does not seem helpful to him, but it came with the promise that God would do just that: help him! Many people who are used victoriously in ministry have been given the thorn that may seem like branding. It is actually a mark of God's sufficient power in their lives.

I will never forget the first time I went to see evangelist and author Nick Vujicic. His message was motivational, but watching him navigate the stage made an even greater impact. He was born without any limbs, and his testimony of joyful perseverance through Christ has made him a powerful witness for the Lord. Nick is a living example of God's strength and grace during challenges.

Joni Eareckson Tada was seventeen years old when she took the dive that left her paralyzed from the neck down. In the years since her accident, her faith and work for the Lord have influenced generations of people across the globe. Her international ministry, Joni and Friends, provides meaningful support and gospel hope to those with disabilities. Joni's honesty about her physical hardships and battles with depression points those with similar afflictions to the hope found in Christ.

The apostle Paul dedicated his life to sharing the good news of salvation through Jesus Christ. God had enabled him to heal others, but when he was tormented by a thorn in his flesh, his repeated prayers were not answered by miraculous healing. Instead, the Lord told him, "My grace is sufficient for you, for my power is made perfect in weakness" (2 Corinthians 12:9).

Have you felt as though your medical condition brands you? Remember that God has great favor and kindness toward you, so do not let health issues become the barometer by which you measure His favor in your life. The miraculous gift of His sufficient help provides us with everything we need to endure any trial. Illness may seem like an ever-present weakness, but it can become a means by which His power is continually at work within us. We may feel branded by our health issues and the limitations they cause, but when we rely on God, we instead bear the imprint of His faithfulness and power. Our lives become rebranded by His sufficient grace.

Pray: Dear God, You are sufficient for all my needs. I know You are willing and able to help me. Your power is more than enough for any weakness or trial I may experience. May my life be a testimony to Your sustaining grace. Give me opportunities to boldly share Jesus, the source of my hope and true strength. In His name I pray. Amen.

Embrace: My weakness is an opportunity to bear a greater imprint of God's faithfulness and power.

Ponder: Have you ever felt branded by suffering or illness? Do you allow illness to leave an imprint of despair on yourself and others? Ask God to rebrand your life so your weakness will display His mighty strength.

Worship: "You Lift Us Up" by Paul Baloche

Homebound

Turn to me and be gracious to me, for I am lonely and afflicted.
—*Psalm 25:16*

Never underestimate the power of one visit.
That flash of recognition,
The instant crinkle of eyes,
An immediate curving smile
That cradles the one
To whom it is offered.
Never underestimate the power of human connection.
Seeing a face you hold dear,
Being seen by someone who cares—
These are a morsel of life to
Someone who is starved for it.
Never underestimate the power of utter isolation,
Of sickness and disease,
Of friends who have moved on,
"Too busy" in their healthy lives.
The isolation wears. And wears. And wears.
The walls of a home are not the only walls for those who are truly alone.
Please visit.

I wrote this poem during one of the most difficult years of my life. Years later, my pastor shared "Homebound" during a sermon series. He read it to encourage our congregation to visit those who are alone or afflicted by health issues. God redeemed my season of loneliness by transforming my expression of pain into a blessing for others who suffer.

In his gospel, Matthew recorded these words from Jesus:

"I was hungry and you gave Me food; I was thirsty and you gave Me drink; I was a stranger and you took Me in; I was naked and you clothed Me; I was sick and you visited Me; I was in prison and you came to Me."

Then the righteous will answer Him, saying, "Lord, when did we see You hungry and feed You, or thirsty and give You drink? When did we see You a stranger and take You in, or naked and clothe You? Or when did we see You sick, or in prison, and come to you?" And the King will answer and say to them, "Assuredly, I say to you, inasmuch as you did it to one of the least of these My brethren, you did it to Me." (25:35–40, NKJV)

Whoever visits, takes care of, or helps meet the needs of those who belong to Christ is serving Jesus Christ Himself. God is concerned about the imprisoned, sick, and needy. He has compassion on those who suffer. Are you isolated or lonely because of your health issues? Please know that being isolated or feeling lonely does not reflect on your value or position as a beloved child of God. Perhaps you can reach out to a family member, friend, local church, or senior center and ask someone to visit you. The visit will bless both of you.

Pray: Jesus, You have such compassion for those who suffer. Thank You for Your command for us to help those in need. Please give me the courage to reach out to others when I am isolated and feeling lonely. Send someone to encourage me and remind me that I am loved. In Your name, amen.

Embrace: Being isolated or feeling lonely does not reflect on my value or position as a beloved child of God.

Ponder: Has the isolation of illness caused you to feel the sting of loneliness? What is one way you can connect with someone today?

Worship: "My Prayer for You" by Alisa Turner

You Have Tremendous Worth

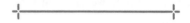

When I consider your heavens, the work of your fingers, the moon and the stars, which you have set in place, what is mankind that you are mindful of them, human beings that you care for them? You have made them a little lower than the angels and crowned them with glory and honor.

—*Psalm 8:3–5*

A Stradivarius violin may have a broken string, sing out of tune, or be played by someone who does not know how to play it, but it will still be worth a great deal. It is, after all, a Stradivarius.

A home designed by Frank Lloyd Wright might need repairs. The wood might rot. The floors might be stained and dirty. The plumbing might need to be fixed. Yet it is still highly regarded. It is, after all, a Frank Lloyd Wright.

A painting or sculpture by Leonardo da Vinci might be plastered with dirt. It can develop cracks or have years of candle soot covering it. A team of highly qualified experts may need to restore its previous beauty. Years of improper treatment may alter its condition but not its importance. It is still, after all, a Leonardo.

You may have been mistreated by those who do not know your true worth. You might need some repairs or have some changes to make to your current condition. Pain and illness might make you feel broken, out of tune, and unable to sing. But nothing—no, not anything—can diminish your value. The apostle Paul was "convinced that neither death nor life, neither angels nor demons, neither the present nor the future, nor any powers, neither height nor depth, nor anything else in all creation, will be able to separate us from the love of God that is in Christ Jesus our Lord" (Romans 8:38–39). You are still, after all, God's beloved creation.

In his devotional *I Lift Up My Soul,* Charles Stanley wrote, "A Stradivarius is valuable because of its maker. We are worthy because God is our Maker. God not only created us; He treasured us enough to make us in His image."[7] Remember who you are by remembering *whose* you are. Illness may have changed your life tremendously, but nothing can change the tremendous worth imparted to you by God.

Pray: Dear God, I confess that I often confuse my abilities and accomplishments with my significance as a person. Please remind me, in those moments, of the incredible worth You imparted to me when You created me. Help me see myself through Your eyes when I feel without purpose, broken down, or worthless because of my infirmities. Thank You for making me in Your image and redeeming me through Jesus Christ. In Jesus's name, amen.

Embrace: Illness may have changed my life tremendously, but nothing can change the tremendous worth imparted to me by God.

Ponder: If your illness has decreased your ability to work or perform daily tasks, how has this affected you? Do you struggle with feelings of low self-worth as a result? How would you encourage a loved one who suffers from illness? How can you receive that advice for yourself?

Worship: "You Say" by Lauren Daigle

Fellow Travelers

Share each other's burdens, and in this way obey the law of
Christ.

—*Galatians 6:2, NLT*

A decade ago, I met a woman who had graduated from my high
school in Florida. That might not seem extraordinary, but we
were both tourists on a whale-watching boat in California! We felt
instant camaraderie as we recounted memories of our school and the
friends we had in common. It is the same when I meet others who
suffer from chronic pain or illness. When you have lived in the life-
changing land of disease, it is easy to bond with others who have
lived there too.

When you are traveling and notice someone with your state flag or
college symbol on their shirt, do you feel an immediate connection?
(You will if you are a Texan. Or if you are my family. No matter where
we travel, they will all yell, "Hook 'em!" to anyone wearing a University of Texas shirt.) Those of us who have lived through illness have
our symbols too. My walker, scooter, and chemo port have inspired
instant connection. I have collected a small group of fellow travelers
this way. I am just as eager to connect with them as they are to connect with me.

When your world has diminished to the four walls of your doctors' offices, your bedroom, or your hospital room, you must find
ways to open those walls and invite others inside. Technology helps
us reach out of our confinement and into the world of someone else
who is confined. We can offer encouragement to one another through
emails, texts, and phone calls. We can look beyond our walls when we

imagine a friend gaining strength from our encouragement. Your impact can reach beyond the confines of your home even if you cannot leave it.

You may be traveling through some lonely places because of illness, but you do not have to do so without meeting a few companions. The Bible says that Jesus often visited lonely places to pray (see Mark 1:45; Luke 5:16). I often wonder who He may have met there, because my lonely places have led me to some remarkable fellow travelers.

Pray: Dear God, I confess that sometimes I feel so alone in my health struggles. Please open my eyes to the suffering of those I meet; let me encourage them with the encouragement You have given me. Please give me courage when I am afraid to reach out to others. Teach me how to support other people who are suffering. Help me recognize that sharing someone's burden may also lift the weight of my own burden. In Jesus's name I pray. Amen.

Embrace: The Lord can help me reach out of my confinement and into the world of someone else who is confined.

Ponder: Do you worry that connecting with someone else who is experiencing illness will be too much of a burden for you to bear? How can you bear others' burdens without sinking under their weight?

Worship: "Love Will Be Our Home" by Sandi Patty

A Fabulous Feast

This final section presents the longest devotionals. Each stand-alone chapter might be just the right choice when you are lonely and want the extra comfort of an extended quiet time.

You **prepare a feast** for me in the *presence of* my enemies.

You honor me by ANOINTING MY HEAD with oil. My cup overflows with blessings.

—Psalm 23:5, NLT

Stop, Look, and Listen

———————————

Whatever is true, whatever is noble, whatever is right, whatever is pure, whatever is lovely, whatever is admirable—if anything is excellent or praiseworthy—think about such things. Whatever you have learned or received or heard from me, or seen in me—put it into practice. And the God of peace will be with you.
—*Philippians 4:8–9*

The classic devotional *Joy and Strength* exhorts us, "One thing is indisputable: the chronic mood of looking longingly at what we have not, or thankfully at what we have, realizes two very different types of character. And we certainly can encourage the one or the other."[1]

Your mind is a powerful God-given tool. Negative thoughts will determine your attitude, and a negative attitude coupled with relentless pain only adds fuel to the fires of despair. You have been given the gift of choice. You can choose how you will respond to the very real frustrations and limitations of illness. Choose to cultivate a thankful spirit by deciding to *stop, look,* and *listen.*

Stop the negative thought in its tracks. When you wake up in pain, unbidden grumbling can float to the surface of your thoughts. Instead of grabbing on to grumbling and letting it carry you through your day, decide that you will hold fast to something else. Begin holding on to God by praying, "I feel the crushing blow of burning pain. It is difficult to get out of bed. Please give me the strength that I need to rise. Lord, I thank You for a new day with new blessings ahead of me. Ready my heart for the good that You are bringing me today."

Look around for your blessings and thank God for them. If you cannot think of any, perhaps the underlying issue is a lack of gratitude. Thankfulness may come more easily to others, but I have to make a conscious effort to thank God when I am in the midst of tough times. Everyone knows people who complain even when their lives are free of significant concerns. You can quietly lead by example when you share the ways God is blessing you during the difficulties of illness.

Listen to truth in Scripture-filled worship songs that build your faith. Fill your ears with praise music and fill your thoughts with gratitude. Sing praises aloud even on days when you do not feel like singing. Building a spiritual life that is rich in thanksgiving can feel like strengthening a muscle. It takes work, but the benefits are worth it. So, keep offering your gratitude to God. Discipline yourself to cultivate thoughts that are life-giving and nurturing to your spirit. It is never too late to start. Thankful thoughts are the bricks that build the foundation of a joy-filled life.

Pray: Dear God, I confess that grumbling about my hardships seems so fitting and natural that I often do not feel like I have a choice in the matter. Help me recognize that my tendency toward complaining will always lead to hopelessness. You have given me self-control, so help me use it. Taming my thoughts becomes easier when I bring praise and thanksgiving into them. Taming my tongue becomes easier when I speak Your praises. Help me obey so that I will be strengthened in You instead of weakened by my complaining spirit. In Jesus's name, amen.

Embrace: Thankful thoughts are the bricks that build the foundation of a joy-filled life.

Practice: Gratitude is a muscle that becomes stronger when you use it. Make a gratitude list, and keep it where you can read over it and give thanks on challenging days. You might not *feel* like giving thanks when you start this practice, but thanksgiving and rejoicing in the Lord always lead to joy that strengthens.

Worship: "Never Stop Singing" by Cross Point Music, featuring Stefan Cashwell

The Father's Gifts

If you sinful people know how to give good gifts to your children, how much more will your heavenly Father give good gifts to those who ask him.
—*Matthew 7:11, NLT*

Jesus taught that the first shall be last and the last shall be first. He said that the meek, not the bold, will inherit the earth. Why are we so surprised when God's gifts for us come through hardship or trial?

I spent many years with complex regional pain syndrome (CRPS) in severe pain and mostly bedridden. Being homebound because of illness is extremely isolating. I grieved over friendships that vanished when my good health began to disappear. Eventually, I found myself living in the lonely kingdom of the homebound. This land seemed to cloak its citizens with invisibility, pain, and suffering that could be seen only by those who also lived there. But I rarely met them because the irony of belonging to this world is that you must be isolated by illness to join. So, alone within the four walls of my bedroom, my constant prayer was this: "God, bring me people who will visit me and not give up on me." Finally, at long last, my prayer became "Jesus, show me Yourself amid all this. Be enough for me. Be present, like a friend to me, in this lonely bedroom."

God answered my prayers in reverse. Jesus did become a very real friend to me; I felt His presence strongly at times. He was the only one who truly knew the depths of my pain, and He was the only one who was awake with me during all my sleepless nights. God also answered my prayers for friendship and support, but the vehicle He used to answer them was a complete shock: I received the diagnosis of another illness. Just like a child opening a present of socks on Christmas, I was thoroughly dismayed and wanted to give it right back. And just like that same child putting on those warm socks on a cold night, I was finally able to derive comfort *through* it, regardless of my disappointment at having received it.

My new diagnosis? Cancer. An aggressive form of non-Hodgkin lymphoma opened the floodgates for channels of love and support to enter my life. Friends who I had not seen in years began to visit. New friends drove me to my chemotherapy sessions. The body of Christ started to uphold me in a way that had mostly eluded me with my other diagnosis. Would I have chosen cancer as a means to restore friendships and bring much-needed fellowship into my life? Absolutely not! But God chose to allow it, and He brought the beautiful gift of loving support alongside it.

Illness never looks like a gift. It looks like pain. It looks like loneliness, fear, and desperation. But we have a Savior who suffered before us and triumphed over it. He promises to walk with us in the darkest valley; His goodness and mercy will pursue us all our days. Our triumphant and faithful God knows our heart's desires. What if the way He chooses to bring them to fruition is difficult? What if our Father's gifts come to us by way of our suffering and pain? In her book *Rose from Brier*, Amy Carmichael said, "I think our Father, who does often give us the pleasure of receiving our heart's desire most beautifully wrapped up, must watch with special love in His eyes when His gifts come in common brown paper, apparently rather badly packed. Shall we find the precious things folded up inside, or shall we be put off?"[2]

Are you able to see any of the gifts that God has given you alongside the pain and struggle of illness? Sometimes you have to look very hard to see them. Often bitterness and resentment harden our hearts to the blessings that come despite—and sometimes because of—our illness. But it is foolish not to embrace the gifts that have come through our trials. They are hard-won and ours for the taking!

Are you bogged down by the burdens that arrive with a difficult diagnosis? Are you grieving the life you once led? It is easy to focus on all that illness has taken from you, but lift your eyes higher. There is a God above who promises to "bless you abundantly, so that in all things at all times, having all that you need, you will abound in every good work" (2 Corinthians 9:8). He is a generous God who delights in giving good gifts to us. He does not wait until our lives are seemingly perfect to send His gifts, as though they were payment or reward. A gift is just that: a gift. And God sends special gifts during—and through—our pain and suffering. Think of Paul pleading with Him to remove the thorn in his flesh. What was God's response to this pleading? He said, "My grace is sufficient for you, for my power is made perfect in weakness" (2 Corinthians 12:9). God's gracious gift to Paul was His perfect power, made manifest despite and because of the weakness of Paul's flesh. The same power is available to us today.

I can relate to Paul. I have prayed many times for healing from my chronic pain, as has my entire family. My son used to ask why God had not healed me when so many people were praying for my healing. But I have come to realize that the greater miracle is that I am a living testimony to God's power. In my weakness and pain, He has sustained me by giving me a faith that can see beyond my present circumstances. I have spent the past twenty years in chronic pain, developed advanced-stage cancer twice, and endured countless surgical procedures. Yet I am smiling as I write this, because I have experienced the greatest miracle of all: joy despite every circumstance. I do not have to manufacture joy; it arrives as beautiful evidence of God's Spirit inside me. Even in my great weakness, I feel His strength propelling me through every crisis. I have experienced God. And He is good.

Pray: God, I confess that I do not always see the gifts that You have for me when I am suffering. Open the eyes of my heart to see all Your abundant goodness in this place of pain and illness. Remind me that I must first offer You the ashes if I am to have beauty for ashes. Take my brokenness and the lost hopes I had for my life. I trust that, in Your time, You will bring beauty from them. Right now, I open my arms to receive all the gifts You want to give me in my suffering. Amen.

Embrace: God sends special gifts during—and through— my pain and suffering.

Practice: Write down the desires of your heart. Commit them to God in prayer, trusting that the Giver of good gifts knows just when and how to give them.

Worship: "Wonder" by Travis Greene, featuring Le'Andria Johnson

Flying into Freedom

Ask where the good way is, and walk in it, and you will find rest for your souls.

—*Jeremiah 6:16*

One thing is more annoying than a fly buzzing in a quiet room, and that is the agitated buzzing of a *trapped* fly. I made this discovery after I mistakenly left a door open and a summer's bounty of insects invaded our home. A lone fly found its way to the room where I read the Bible, write, and spend time with the Lord. My quiet sanctuary is no place for a loudly buzzing insect!

I heard the fly late at night, and it was buzzing just as loudly and frantically the following day. The poor creature seemed caught in the space between our windowpane and our wide venetian blinds. The blinds were completely open to the room, so there were twenty-one sizable spaces (I counted!) that offered true freedom to this pitiful insect. But for an entire day, it was focused on trying to escape back into the familiar outside world. Since the exit to the outdoors was covered by glass, it offered no freedom at all.

How often do I do the same thing? Like Eve before me, I want the one thing that I am denied. I look out at the lives of others—so full of activities, people, and places—yet the windowpane of disease keeps that world from me. Just like the fly, I make frantic attempts to break through the glass. My body hits it at full force when I schedule activities and make demands of myself that my body cannot manage. I will always end up worn out, in pain, and mightily discouraged. Other times, beset by frustration and self-pity, I huddle on the windowsill between both worlds and give up trying to break through anything at all.

Wretched fly that I am! If I would quit buzzing around and simply rest for a moment, I might hear a quiet voice guiding me to greater freedom. After all, even the fly was not truly trapped. The open blinds that offered an escape may have looked disappointing compared with the world beyond the window, as they lead into my home instead of into the sunny outdoors. But there is freedom in going in the direction God has made available to you.

I might not like having to stay home when pain or disease limits my activities, but there are ways that I can still function. There are ways that I can still have a rich and full life if I would only look around for them. I will pray for the perspective to find the paths that are open to me. Then I will soar through them and joyfully embrace my freedom.

Pray: Dear God, I confess that I often do not like the limitations or side effects of my illness, pain, medications, and disabilities. They are genuine hardships for me. I know that You created me and that Your plans for my life are good. Help me find new ways to be active and connect with others. Open the door to creative endeavors. Open the door to greater fellowship. Open my heart to receive everything You have for me. Change my perspective, and help me embrace that Your plan is better than I could have ever imagined. In Jesus's powerful name, amen.

Embrace: There is freedom in going in the direction God has made available to me.

Practice: If illness prevents you from living the life you used to live, then ask God to show you the areas that are still open to you. Pray for Him to provide new activities, ministries, or other avenues that will bring joy and fulfillment back into your life.

Worship: "Worn" by Tenth Avenue North

The Princess

All glorious is the princess within her chamber; her gown is interwoven with gold. In embroidered garments she is led to the king; her virgin companions follow her—those brought to be with her. Led in with joy and gladness, they enter the palace of the king.

—*Psalm 45:13–15*

I spent my week enduring infusion procedures for pain, and my vanity has attended every appointment. Having to spend hours each day with my mind numbed by chemicals made me feel like I was dying a mini death every time, yet I clung fastidiously to trappings of comeliness. I wore lipstick, fixed my hair, and donned clothing that would be stylish yet comfortable to sleep in during the five hours of daily infusions. All was vanity. I was actually just lying down and receiving an infusion that temporarily suspended my thoughts and memories in the desperate hope of numbing my pain. To avoid losing myself completely, I did all I could to ensure that the body lying on the treatment table resembled the person I used to be.

During one such infusion, I overheard one of the nurses say to my nurse, "How is the little princess today?" Perhaps she thought I could not hear her as I lay silent on the table. Maybe she was speaking about someone else, but a gut instinct told me that she was talking about me. It could have been a kind term of affection. It might have been a biting commentary on how she perceived me. I will never know. Even in the medicine-induced haze of my infusion, something about the phrase grabbed my attention because this was not the first time someone had called me a little princess.

When I was a young child, my grandmother was the person I most wanted to please. I treasured everything she said to me; her compliments lifted me, and her criticisms sharply deflated me. Grandma always called me her little princess, and my heart would soar with this term of endearment. It meant that I was special, set apart, and loved. I fully believed, at age four, that I was indeed a princess, whatever that meant.

One day, at a White Castle restaurant in Ohio, my grandmother told me it was the perfect place for me to eat since I was her little princess. I finally asked her, "Grandma, what *is* a princess?" Her explanation that a princess was a daughter of a king or queen and that I was not really a princess came as a shock to me. I remember sitting at that table, waiting for the square hamburger with the squishy bread that White Castle is famous for, devastated to learn that I was not a princess after all.

How many people can say they distinctly recall the day they discovered they were not royalty? I can laugh about it now. But at age four, I was mortified to learn that princesses did, in fact, exist but that I was not one of them. It is entirely possible that tears were shed. This revelation took all my unrecognized yet deeply held beliefs about myself and pulled them out from under me in a heartbeat: I was no longer special since I was not a princess. In the years that followed, I tried everything I could think of to reclaim my royal status, but I learned the hard way that vanity and perfectionism are not paths to the palace.

After the nurse's remark, I wrote the following in my journal:

So now here I am. The little princess. Sleeping Beauty Princess, lying on a cold metal table with IV tubing delivering a cocktail of mind-altering drugs for hours on end. Long hair flowing over a pillow brought from the home she desperately wants to return to and be able to take care of once again. Cinderella Princess, who cannot dance at the ball but cannot clean the fireplace in her rags either. Snow White Princess, with red lipstick crusted around dry lips that slowly take in oxygen supplied by the cold plastic mask. Eyes flicker open for a moment, struggling to understand where she is and what is happening to her, both mind and memory saturated with poison from this apple she has chosen to bite. Hands stiff and unmoving, clawing the soft blanket brought for comfort and warmth. Flesh and bones are lying still, soaking up the potion that promises not youth, not beauty, but simply offering a chance to be free. Free of pain. Free of gnarled hands and limping gait. I have become the Princess of Pain, hovering over midnight, my happily ever after in another land.

Every fairy tale has defining moments. Sometimes a kiss from a prince transforms a princess and ushers her into her happily ever after. I can patiently await my moment because my prince is waiting for me too. His name is Jesus. He is the Prince of Peace, bringing peace with God to all who call on His name. In obedience to God, He stepped down from His throne and gave His life to purchase all of us, even though we are imprisoned by sin and death. Imagine, the life of the Prince given for a prisoner! But the story is not over. Jesus was raised to life again, and all those who call on His name will enter His kingdom. It only *seems* too good to be true. It is, in fact, history. And it is also my future.

One day this broken body will be totally transformed and fit for life in the new kingdom. I will be clothed with immortality that devours all pain and disease and tears and sorrow and death. Pain will not escape! Illness will not escape! They will be completely conquered. Forever. For now, my body feels the curse of this present kingdom. But one day I will enter an eternal kingdom, ruled by the One who had no beauty or majesty to attract but who is Beauty and Majesty itself. He is the Prince of Peace and the King of kings. He has loved me with an everlasting love and chosen me as His bride, so I am a princess after all—not by anything I have done but by all He has done for me. I am loved by Him and redeemed by Him, and I will spend eternity with Him. I will have my happily ever after at last.

Pray: Dear God, sometimes the ravages of illness affect how I see myself. Help me see me as You see me; I am the child of the King. Let the beauty of Jesus shine so brightly in me that it is the first thing people notice when they look at me. Help me wear my outward signs of illness as a badge of all You are helping me overcome. Thank You for the hope of eternal healing and redemption that is mine in the Prince of Peace and King of kings. I love You. Thank You for preparing a place for me in the palace. In Jesus's precious name I pray. Amen.

Embrace: Jesus is preparing a place in the palace just for me.

Ponder: Are you similarly assured of having a happily ever after? Why or why not? In what ways does the promise of redemption and healing give you strength to endure?

Worship: "Revelation Song" by Michael W. Smith

Truth That Keeps Me from Faltering

It is God who works in you to will and to act in order to fulfill his good purpose.

—Philippians 2:13

I recently came across this old journal entry:

I dreamed last night that I was walking with a rubber band around my feet: faltering steps and pain around my ankles with each motion. When I awoke, my muscles felt tired and worn-out, proof of my nighttime escapades. This dream was no mistake. My illness binds me and causes me to walk at a different pace, both literally and figuratively. In the dream, I was embarrassed and assumed that others around me must wonder why I don't just take off the rubber band.

I feel like that in real life as well. My journal entry continued:

When people's comments reveal that they think I should just "get on with" my life and throw off the rubber bands of pain and fatigue, I am embarrassed and ashamed that I suffer from illness, as if it is an act of will to be healed or a choice that someone who is "stronger" would make.

The Bible is such a comfort to me when I am having

thoughts like this. There are so many examples of
people who suffered from pain and disease. Jesus never
said to any of them, "Just get over it, exercise more,
stop thinking about your pain, and you will be better!"
I hunger for His healing in my life. But most of all,
I long for God to be glorified through me.

I once met a health writer at a Christian conference. This man had written a book about what he felt were biblical solutions for disease. I was amazed to read that he thought anger and an unforgiving spirit were the causes of chronic pain and disease. He surmised that illness was a direct punishment for sin. How did Jesus respond to a similar misconception when His disciples asked whose sin was responsible for a man's blindness? Jesus said, "Neither this man nor his parents sinned . . . but this happened so that the works of God might be displayed in him" (John 9:3). He was not suggesting that the man and his parents were not sinners. Instead, He corrected the disciples in their mistaken belief that the man's physical ailment was a punishment for or result of sin. Jesus taught the disciples, and all of us who read the account, that there is a higher purpose behind physical affliction.

I do not know what causes chronic pain or disease. I do know, however, that there are plenty of angry and unforgiving people who do not have chronic pain. I also know that many who suffer from disease are gentle and merciful individuals. Perhaps our sovereign God allowed suffering so He could display His tremendous power through us. I am learning to live, not despite pain or disease but by accepting them as part of what God will use in my life to accomplish His purposes. German poet Georg Neumark wrote a wonderful poem that speaks to this. Since he wrote it in the 1600s, it reminds us that the struggle to accept difficult circumstances has been present through the ages.

Only be still, and wait His leisure
In cheerful hope, with heart content
To take whate'er thy Father's pleasure,
And all-discerning love hath sent;
Nor doubt our inmost wants are known
To Him who chose us for His own.[3]

God knows your innermost wants, and He has intentionally sifted every circumstance in your life through His very loving hands. There is a purpose in your pain, and it is not despair! Let your pain guide you to His arms, and trust that your creator knows your deepest desires. After all, "in all things God works for the good of those who love him, who have been called according to his purpose" (Romans 8:28). God will use every circumstance to work good in our lives. When trials lead me to question my faith, these two truths restore it: God is sovereign, and God is good. Since this is so, I can trust Him even when illness makes life difficult to bear.

Pray: Jesus, let Your glory be revealed in my life amid my brokenness, my pain, and the rubber bands of insufficiency. Stretch the cords that are holding me back and causing my steps to falter. Be my strength, and enable me to walk Your path daily. In Your name I pray. Amen.

Embrace: God is sovereign, and God is good. I can trust Him even when illness makes life difficult to bear.

Ponder: Have you ever had someone tell you that your illness is a result of your sin? Sometimes, even in their efforts to help, people can say things that wound us. Have you forgiven this person? Your health issues are heavy enough; carry the weight of this offense to the Lord, and discover the freedom of *choosing* to forgive.

Worship: "Even If" by MercyMe

My Power Source

Do you not know? Have you not heard? The LORD is the everlasting God, the Creator of the ends of the earth. He will not grow tired or weary, and his understanding no one can fathom. He gives strength to the weary and increases the power of the weak.
—*Isaiah 40:28–29*

When visiting family in Florida, I decided to take my three children to Disney World. I wanted their childhoods to be filled with joyful memories and the knowledge that, despite being ill, their mom did all she could for them. You may wonder how someone with chronic pain can manage to visit Disney World. I have three words for you: electric conveyance vehicle (ECV), otherwise known as a mobility scooter.

The ECV is a blessing for those of us who cannot manage to walk for hours on end. I used it frequently throughout the long days in the theme park, walking for a bit when my back hurt from sitting. I was so grateful to have a device that enabled me to enjoy Disney World with my children. However, I was very aware of the looks that others gave me; some looked with curiosity and others looked with pity. Many looked with anger because of the extra time it took me to drive up a ramp on the resort bus. I was ashamed of my need.

One day, while sitting on the monorail in the ECV, I felt incredibly vulnerable and sensitive to the stares of those around me. Suddenly a Bible verse I had memorized years before came to my mind: "He gives strength to the weary and increases the power of the weak" (Isaiah 40:29). The Lord spoke to my heart, saying, *I am increasing your power. You cannot walk this park in your own strength, but I have provided the power for you to manage it.* I sat up in the cart, feeling so blessed that the Lord allowed me to have this external power source. I met curious stares with a joyful smile because I no longer felt ashamed of my need. Instead, I felt grateful for my provision.

Where is God providing strength in your life? Perhaps He has given you people who help you perform daily tasks. Maybe He has allowed you to listen to a sermon on the television or computer when illness prevents you from attending church. God brings power into our lives in so many ways. I will always ask Him to increase my strength during illness, but now I will also notice the areas in which He has already provided it. Whether our Father uses an external power source such as an ECV or provides me with internal power to withstand my painful struggles, He does indeed give strength to the weary and increase the power of the weak.

Pray: Dear God, You have given me the power to navigate the difficulties of illness. Thank You for all the ways You strengthen and revive me. Even when I am physically weak and fatigued, You strengthen my spirit so I can withstand my temporary afflictions. Please open my eyes so I can truly see all the ways You provide for me, strengthen me, and give me the power to overcome my challenges. Help me rely on You. Thank You for caring about me. Amen.

Embrace: When I am grateful for my provision, I will no longer feel ashamed of my need.

Practice: In what ways does God help you when you are worn out by illness? Can you name someone or something that helps you during your battle with health issues? Have you thanked God for that person or thing? Take some time to thank Him for all the ways He provides for your needs.

Worship: "You Are My Strength" by William Murphy

The Key to All Treasure

I will give you the treasures of darkness and hidden riches of secret places.

—Isaiah 45:3, NKJV

More than a decade ago, I wrote the following in my journal:

Do not fear the valley of the shadow, or run from it, or you will miss the beautiful treasures that can be found here. The enemy of your soul would love to chase you from them. He uses fear and constant preoccupation with the dark shadowlands of trial and tribulation to turn your eyes away from the precious gems that are within your reach. Satan wants to trap you with keys of hopelessness, self-pity, and despair, and then he uses those keys to lock you into his chains of defeat. Do not be deceived. These are not the keys that will open the treasure vaults of God.

God prompted me with a thought about how to break the chains of defeat by seeking a victorious life in Christ. I continued in my journal:

The keys of the enemy lead to death: death of joy, death of hope, and death of faith. The enemy does not want you to find God's treasures, because they will

*mightily empower you and equip you for the victory
of living an abundant life in Christ.*

If you knew where to find unimaginable treasure and someone told you what you needed to do to find the key to unlock it, what would you do? What if you could fully access the treasure even from your sickbed, hospital room, workplace, or home? You have an invitation to a storehouse of blessing that is not limited to the healthy and able-bodied! The key to God's treasure is proper fear of and reverence for the Lord. When you worship Him during your trials, even the darkest night cannot hide the treasure He has placed there for you to discover.

Fearing the Lord is like having a dual-purpose key. It simultaneously turns the lock to free us from the chains that bind us and opens the treasure that God wants to give us. I have experienced it. When pain has so utterly consumed me that I thought I could not live another moment in its grasp, I determinedly sought the Lord through praise and thanksgiving. It took discipline for me to drop despair and pick up a key of praise, but honoring Him this way brings us freedom. Praise unlocked strength and perseverance; these beautiful treasures helped me through this particular darkness. We should never fear entering the dark places in our lives when we have a Lord who has entered them first and bestows His gifts of victory on those who follow Him there.

You have been given a key. What will you do with it?

Pray: Lord, forgive me when I turn my attention away from You and become entrapped by self-pity and despair. Show me the keys I have been using lately; take away any that are not of You. You alone are God, so let the weight of Your authority in my life cause me to humbly bow in worship and rise in joy. I leave all my desires, hopes, worries, and hardships—my entire life—at the foot of Your throne. May the light of Your presence illuminate the treasures You have for me in my present darkness. In Jesus's name, amen.

Embrace: Fearing the Lord is like having a dual-purpose key that frees me from bondage and opens the treasure that God wants to give me.

Ponder: "He will be the sure foundation for your times, a rich store of salvation and wisdom and knowledge; the fear of the LORD is the key to this treasure" (Isaiah 33:6). What do you think "the fear of the LORD" means? How can it be a key that unlocks treasure? What treasure do you think you will find there? Is it worth pursuing?

Worship: "Restored (The Grindstone Song)" by Cheri Keaggy

The Garden of Solitude

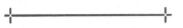

I will make an everlasting covenant with them: I will never stop doing good for them. I will put a desire in their hearts to worship me, and they will never leave me. I will find joy doing good for them and will faithfully and wholeheartedly replant them in this land.

—*Jeremiah 32:40–41, NLT*

I wrote this entry in my journal when I was entirely homebound:

My current growing season has been exceedingly painful, but the Master Gardener knows what I need to thrive. When a plant has become root-bound, a caring gardener disengages it from its container. The roots must be broken apart, and the plant must be replanted in a place where it can have room to spread out. It seems as though God has broken through some of my roots; He is using illness to rake apart my life. He has replanted me in a different part of His garden, away from the foot traffic. He knows what I need to grow and thrive, how much shade or heat I need, and how much pruning I must endure to be fruitful.

Before I became disabled by illness, I taught elementary school and led Bible studies, Mothers of Preschoolers (MOPS) groups, and even the occasional workshop. Conducting workshops and teaching brought joy and excitement because I love interacting with people.

Now, because of illness, I am homebound. I miss teaching. I miss people. But it seems that God has a reason for replanting me in solitude; He is calling me to develop something other than loneliness. I am called to develop something that will encourage others. I am called to write. I used to wonder how I would ever fulfill that calling. Whenever I wrote a story or devotional, friends and family encouraged me to keep writing. But I would make excuses because I did not want to cultivate the solitude necessary to do it. Being around people inspired and recharged me; sitting alone to write was not appealing in the least. Then came illness.

I am always inspired by authors who write amid health issues or other suffering. Here are three examples that readily come to mind:

Missionary Amy Carmichael is well known for her ministry to children in India. She authored many books, even managing to write one while bedridden with pain. Reading *Rose from Brier* brought great encouragement to me when I was first learning to live with the severe pain of CRPS, because Miss Carmichael had the exact symptoms and disease course I have. I am convinced that she also lived with CRPS, although I cannot find any record of her having received that diagnosis since it was not as understood in the early 1900s as it is today. I will always be grateful that she used the time her illness gave her to write this book, as her words of encouragement still speak today.

King David used times of solitude and hiding (even in a cave!) to write out his cries of desperation to God. He poured his faith, praise, turmoil, and pain into songs and onto the page. David's writings are part of God's Word for a reason! What believer has not benefited from these psalms? Even those who do not believe are comforted by them. The psalms have such power to bring us hope and encouragement. None of his suffering was in vain.

Finally, Jean-Dominique Bauby, a French journalist with the condition called locked-in syndrome, had only the movement of his left eyelid. His helpers read a list of letters aloud and watched him blink when they said the precise letter he wanted. Then they wrote down the letter he had chosen. Bauby wrote an entire book, *The Diving Bell and the Butterfly,* by blinking his eye to indicate what he wanted to communicate—letter by letter, word by word, sentence by sentence. His tenacity has inspired me. Surely, even with CRPS in my hands, I can push through my pain and use a pen to write.

God can use our diseases and other hardships to bring about His purposes for our lives in unexpected ways. He uses suffering to plumb the depths of our hearts and rid us of anything that hinders us from completely and unabashedly following Him. God has a purpose for the pain in our lives. He even has a purpose for isolation. In my life, that solitude has allowed me to write. A Bible, a journal, and a pen fill the days I spend alone in my home. In my loneliness of being homebound with illness, Jesus has become my all. Are you isolated by illness? You are not alone in your solitude. God has not forgotten you. Continue abiding in Him so you will flourish wherever He chooses to plant you.

Pray: God, You see all the changes that illness has made in my life. I am no longer able to participate in the activities that seemed to give my life purpose and meaning. Show me that You have given me a purpose and that my life has meaning apart from my accomplishments. Forgive me for the times I turn away from You; help me follow You wholeheartedly. Fill me with Your Holy Spirit, and bring me the comfort of Your love. In Your name I pray. Amen.

Embrace: God has not forgotten me; I will flourish in His care wherever He chooses to plant me.

Practice: Writer Henri Nouwen reflected, "To live a spiritual life we must first find the courage to enter into the desert of loneliness and to change it by gentle and persistent efforts into a garden of solitude."[4] What is the difference between a desert of loneliness and a garden of solitude? Which spiritual practices can create the shift from one to the other? Set aside time for one of those practices this week.

Worship: "There Was Jesus" by Zach Williams and Dolly Parton

Mammon Isn't My Friend

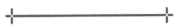

Those who cling to worthless idols turn away from God's love for them.

—*Jonah 2:8*

Author Os Hillman shared this insightful commentary about spending our lives pursuing material objects:

Jesus once said, "No servant can serve two masters.... You cannot serve both God and money" (Luke 16:13). In the original language, the word translated "money" was an Aramaic word, *Mammon*.... The people of Jesus' day thought of Mammon as a false god. Jesus ... said that those who spend their lives seeking worldly gain are idolaters.[5]

When illness causes isolation, we search for anything to quickly fill the aching void. An abundance of possessions can begin to take the place that friends used to occupy. No one is visiting me? It's okay; I have packages from multiple companies coming to my door each day. Admittedly, the thrill of receiving something is often my only excitement these days, but it is a short-lived escape, and I just end up with more stuff. I am always trying to escape my pain and illnesses, yet I am drowning in my escape.

Possessions can seem safer to escape into than friendships because they do not leave you, hurt you, or gossip about you. When health issues begin to keep you at home, some friendships remain in the elusive land of the healthy. Many friends do not want to enter into a world of illness and pain. They might make excuses by telling you that they do not want to bother you and will wait until you feel better to get together. When you have been devastated by chronic illness, wounds like these from friends can be easily magnified and add to the pain of suffering.

Material objects only *seem* safer than relationships. The truth is that things fall out of style, break, become soiled, no longer meet our needs, no longer fit our bodies, and simply do not satisfy. Truly committed friendships can always transform, and God uses these friendships to transform us. They are hard work at times but necessary work if we are to experience the fullness of God's love through them. There is a reason so many Scripture verses are devoted to remaining in the fellowship and unity of a body of other believers. God knows we need one another.

Caring for another, the mutual give-and-take of friendship, seems overwhelming when I am in pain. I don't have the mental or emotional energy to lift up somebody else or think of their problems. It is a tremendous use of psychological energy to analyze facial expressions, words, and the things left unsaid during a conversation. I cannot manage this when pain is screaming in the background and demanding all my attention. It seems easier for me, in my homebound boredom, to focus on things that don't have needs and won't say something that might hurt me and cause me to topple further.

But using material objects in the place that God designed for fellowship with Him and others will not only topple me but also devastate me. Even the most valuable object does not offer the hope and fulfillment that only God can bring, yet I easily buy into the lie that material things will satisfy. The reality is that they just carry the weight of financial debt along with the burden of emptiness. Then they heap on the additional load of more stuff to care for and organize, which steals time and energy that could be spent in fellowship with God and others. The appetite for things is a never-ending hunger that keeps me from the feast. I thought I had power over the possessions that entered my life, but actually they have power over me. They are false gods who entrap and ensnare. They are Mammon.

I can spend my entire life caring for my possessions, but they cannot ever care for me. Lately, I have felt a growing sense of hopelessness. Today I realized I have no hope because my heart is in the hands of the wrong master. "Those who run after other gods will suffer more and more" (Psalm 16:4). Hope is dead when it is wasted on a god who is not God. I am not opening the door to a friend when I welcome Mammon. Instead, I will open my door to true friends, and I will open my heart to the Lord, who is my faithful companion in suffering and my comforter in every sorrow.

Pray: God, thank You for never giving up on me. You see all the ways I dishonor You, yet You are always ready to call me into fellowship with You. You are the Friend who will never leave me. Please help me not show contempt for the riches of Your kindness, forbearance, and patience. Remind me that You are not just my friend but also my master and my king. Forgive me when I exalt anything above You; give me a proper perspective. Draw me close, God; I need You. In the mighty name of Jesus, amen.

Embrace: The appetite for possessions is a never-ending hunger that keeps me from the feast.

Ponder: Have you noticed that you spend time purchasing things you do not need in your efforts to cope with isolation, boredom, or the weight of your diagnosis? If so, how has this helped or hurt you?

Worship: "Better" by Pat Barrett

My Divine Appointment

You will be brought before kings and governors [and doctors and nurses and patients] for my name's sake. This will be your opportunity to bear witness.
*—Luke 21:12–13, ESV, John Piper's words in brackets,
from* Lessons from a Hospital Bed

I received an unexpected letter from MD Anderson Cancer Center a few years ago. The doctor was concerned about my routine mammogram and wanted me to have an ultrasound and core needle biopsy. I could either have it here in Austin or go to MD Anderson in Houston, but further testing is more complicated than it seems. My overactive pain response means that any trauma to my body, such as a biopsy, causes intense burning, viselike crushing, and stabbing pain that typically remains for years. Every surgical procedure or injection must be worth the risk of long-term pain.

Understandably, I was filled with anxiety when I awoke early the day after I received the letter. My husband and I asked God for wisdom. We finished praying together, and I sensed that God was leading me to have the testing at MD Anderson. My husband quietly continued to bow his head in silent prayer. When he finally looked up, he said, "We should just go to Houston."

I thought back to the long medical-center hallways and the sobering days spent in waiting rooms with people who were suffering. I remembered the complete exhaustion of a full day spent enduring testing. And I inwardly protested, *I don't want to have to go back there!* But the Lord spoke to my spirit and said, *How can you minister to people who have health issues if you are not around them?* This gentle rebuke filled me with joy and reminded me of this truth: There is always a greater plan at work.

I realized that God had a purpose in drawing me back there again, and it was not to cause suffering. He had appointments for me, not only with the medical staff but also with other patients and their families. Whenever I go to MD Anderson, other patients openly share their cancer stories and allow me the opportunity to pray with them. In this way, a medical appointment opens the door to ministry that God has appointed.

A few moments after this realization, I flipped open the book *Lessons from a Hospital Bed*, by John Piper, and read these words: "You are nowhere by mere coincidence. . . . These are all divine appointments."[6]

Lord, help me get ready for *all* the appointments You have for me.

Pray: Dear God, I am often so wrapped up in my health battles that I forget to notice others who are suffering. Please help me see those who need Your love. Help me listen to their stories. Give me the courage I need in order to be willing to pray with them. The medical staff also need encouragement, so let me speak Your words as I seek to uplift them. Teach me creative ways to bless those I meet during my appointments. You have a greater purpose, always for good, when You lead me to difficult places. I trust You, God. In Jesus's name, amen.

Embrace: The Great Designer always has a greater design at work.

Ponder: Praying with other people offers a depth of support that is essential when we experience hardship. Do you have anyone who regularly prays with you? If not, why not? If you're not already part of a local Bible-believing church, consider contacting one and asking to be put in touch with someone who will pray for you—or someone for whom you can pray. You could also turn to page 269 in the Resources section for information about a twenty-four-hour prayer hotline.

Worship: "He Leadeth Me" by the Martins

My Visit to the Cancer Center

Like cold water to a weary soul is good news from a distant land.
—*Proverbs 25:25*

I undergo testing a few times a year to monitor my lymph nodes for signs of cancer progression or remission. (Of course I hope and pray for remission!) I wrote the following passage to describe my visit—and my eagerness to hear the good news of cancer remission from my doctor.

Today is the day for my cancer staging. It is the day to find out if the cancer has shrunk, grown, or spread. This is the day for the fasting, the poking, and the prodding. The day for lying in a metal tube, for having my port accessed, for a barium drink, and for contrast dye. This is the day for the automated voice in the CT machine that says, "Take a breath—hold it," and then just when I feel like I will pass out, it finally says, "You can breathe."

This is the day for community, a day to look others in the face and say, "You too?" It is the day to hear stories about surgeries, medicines, and treatment options from perfect strangers and it isn't strange at all because they know I understand. It is the day to be bold, the day to pray with people I meet who I might see again, and the day to pray with those I might never see again on this earth. Ever. It is the day to look directly into the eyes of patients whose bald heads and face masks obscure all but those weary eyes and to communicate that I see past what illness has done to them. I can see because I was once a person with a bald head and face mask with weary eyes pleading, "See *me*." So now I see. And they are beautiful.

This is the day for seemingly endless walking and waiting. Walking and waiting. Walking and waiting. Walking to each new department. Waiting with all the other hopeful people. We hope that the treatment has worked and that cancer has lessened its hold on us. Or we are hoping to find a treatment at all. Streaming through hallways to the next appointment, some of us walk purposefully and seem ready to fight the battle that has come our way. Others are pushed in wheelchairs by those who have taken up the fight with us. And so we walk. And we wait.

Then all the tests are read, from offices and labs that we do not see and by people we do not meet. They are unseen heroes in our battle, working tirelessly around the clock to arm us with the report of the enemy's whereabouts so we can know where to attack. We arrive for the doctor's appointment, ready to hear our battle strategy, preparing ourselves in the only ways we know how. In the vast waiting area, some patients are silently praying. Some are joking and laughing, eager to have a bit of normalcy in a situation that was not the norm they had counted on. Others are reading, trying to escape the realities of the day. But behind closed eyes, behind humorous quips, and behind the covers of a book, we all have this: uncertainty.

When we are finally called back to the doctor's office by a smiling nurse, we feel like runners nearing the finish line of a marathon. At this point, we are so exhausted that we almost forgot why we were running. "Just send me the results," we want to say. "I am going home to sleep the rest of the day." But curiosity gets the best of us—that *and* a desire to live. So we wait for the doctor to give us the results.

This is the moment when all pretense is stripped bare. Whatever the outcome of our tests and lab reports, we cannot stop the flood of feelings that arises upon hearing them. This is often how we realize what our real expectations were. Did we expect to hear worse news, or did we expect news of remission? The truth is revealed in this moment. But it makes no difference. The report is the report, and feelings or previous expectations will not change it.

This is also the moment in time when, if the news is good, we give thanks with relief that we have won the current skirmish. Or we are stunned into temporary defeat when we hear reports about the victory that cancer seems to be gaining over us. One moment to the next can change our entire outlook on life. Yet nothing has changed. It was already growing or it wasn't. The only difference is that now we know what was happening in there. Cancer was continually growing larger in the back of our minds; now we know if it was also growing in our bodies. Now we know.

And now I know. Now I know that the words I hoped to hear were not to be spoken at this visit. The four little words, spoken together, would harmonize into a glorious song of freedom. Or so I imagined. I will write them here, but on paper they lose their power. When they are not truthfully uttered to someone for whom they carry the weight of hopes, the embodiment of prayers, and the earnestness of heartfelt desire, they lose their power. These words were not for me this time, but I write them here for you to see. Notice how flat they are, the words that were unstrung, folded up, and packed back into the doctor's bag for someone else to hear. Here is the symphony of words that remain, for me, just notes on a page:

You are in remission.

Pray: Lord, help me rejoice in You every day You have allotted to me. Give me the faith to trust You on the days that hold difficult news of a crushing diagnosis. It wearies me to undergo testing and procedures, but I recognize that I am blessed to be able to receive medical care. Thank You for all the medical staff who work hard to help me. Please bless those who wait with me at appointments or visit me when I am in the hospital. Give them the peace they need. Give them support, Lord, as they are often weary in a different way. Lift us up, and hold us close to Your heart today. Amen.

Embrace: Only God can carry all my hopes, dreams, and prayers; my doctor's report is too small to hold that much weight.

Practice: You may not have a cancer diagnosis, but everyone with extensive health issues can relate to the experience of visiting medical centers or undergoing tests. Write down a few Bible verses that help your anxiety or fear when you go to the hospital for testing or a medical procedure. Bring them with you to pray over while you are in the waiting room.

Worship: "How Great Thou Art" by Joey + Rory

Say a Prayer, Cut My Hair

Where two or three are gathered in My name [meeting together
as My followers], I am there among them.
—*Matthew 18:20, AMP*

Birthday parties. Weddings. Graduations. Who would have thought that one day we would stop gathering together to celebrate? But that is precisely what happened when COVID arrived in our world. We collectively mourned, and we prayed for the day when we could gather with friends. God made us for fellowship with one another, so we yearned for the gatherings we once took for granted.

Throughout Scripture, we find God-ordained occasions to gather for celebration. We are even invited to a wedding feast in heaven! There is no question that gathering together is important to God. It is also important to me, so I decided to have a "Say a Prayer, Cut My Hair" party when I was about to undergo chemotherapy. I needed the strength and prayer support of my sisters in Christ, so I invited a group of friends over, and each one prayed over me, then cut off a portion of my long hair. It turned losing my hair into a time of great blessing. There were tears. There was laughter. And there is not a single photo from that night where I am not smiling, because I experienced the deep and abiding love of Christ through each one of my beautiful friends.

Every party needs a party favor. Even a "Say a Prayer, Cut My Hair" party. (And no, I did not give my hair away as the favor. I am a better hostess than that!) I contacted a friend who works for a cosmetics firm, and she graciously put together beautiful bags with samples.

I used the name of each item to write tributes to the ladies who attended the party. Gathering with friends to pray and speak words of blessing can turn a difficult time into a memorable moment of celebration.

Here is a list of the skin-care samples and what I typed on a tag attached to them:

Skin Booster: You have each, in different ways, boosted me up when I have been pulled down by pain and circumstance.

Light Eye Mask: You have each helped brighten my eyes and my spirit by bringing the light of Jesus into my world on days when all I could see was darkness.

Response Cream: Thank you for being quick to respond when I ask for help.

Perfume Sample: Proverbs 27:9 says it best: "Oil and perfume make glad the heart, and the wise suggestion of a friend is sweet to the soul." God has used each of you to bring both sweetness and wisdom into my life, and I am thankful.

Eye Cream: This eye cream says it repairs and defends. Each of you has been quick to run to my defense by praying for me. You rally the armies of God on my behalf, and I know you will continue to do so as I walk through this trial with cancer.

Lipstick: Last but not least, because this was a product that I love, I wanted each of you to have "Instant Pick-Me-Up Lips." Every time I talk to or see each of you, it has always been an instant pick-me-up. Thank you so much for being my friends.

Pray: Dear God, thank You that I don't need good news to celebrate, because *You* are the good news! I can celebrate Your goodness and faithfulness even during a life-altering diagnosis.

Thank You for the fellowship of other believers. Help us honor You and encourage one another in Christlikeness. Thank You for teaching us how to love one another. In Jesus's name, amen.

Embrace: Fellowship with other believers strengthens me so I can endure seasons of suffering.

Ponder: A journey through illness is not filled with parties; it is often filled with great isolation. How are you meeting your need for fellowship right now? Can you commit to going to an online Bible study or attending a prayer group? Pray that God would show you how to meet your need for fellowship with other believers.

Worship: "When We Gather" by Brad and Rebekah

The Hidden Cost of Medication

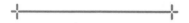

There is now no condemnation for those who are in Christ Jesus.
—*Romans 8:1*

My sixteen-year-old daughter almost ran a minivan off the road, with her little brother in the back seat of our car, as she rushed me to the emergency room. Although I tried to reassure my children that I was probably fine, the fear in their eyes told me they knew otherwise. After all, we'd been about to visit the children's museum that morning when I'd asked my daughter, recently licensed, to drive me to the hospital instead.

The nagging lower abdominal pain I'd had for a month had been excruciating the previous evening, but that morning it had felt better. However, I'd become clammy, dizzy, and nauseated right before we left the house. I tried to lie down for a moment, which then caused sharp pain in my shoulders. Sitting up in bed, I began a slow fade into sleep, until a vision flashed through my mind: *I was lying on the floor outside my bedroom with my children standing, terrified, over my body.* The scene was shocking enough to propel me out of bed and into the car for a trip to the emergency room. My anxiety about being driven by my teenage daughter was only heightened by the prospect of telling hospital staff about my medication.

At that time, I took prescribed pain medication to function with CRPS. Admitting to hospital staff that I took a strong medication with the potential for addiction was embarrassing because I valued living a completely sober lifestyle. Although Scripture clearly allows responsible alcohol use, Paul's admonition in Ephesians 5:18—"Do not get drunk with wine . . . but be filled with the [Holy] Spirit and constantly guided by Him" (AMP)—is a foundational principle in my life. Part of the agony of living with excruciating pain is being so conflicted and embarrassed about taking the only medication that partially alleviates it.

As we pulled up to the hospital, I gave my children money and instructed them to see a movie at the nearby theater while the doctors examined me. The staff immediately led me to the nurses' station when I recounted my symptoms. But as soon as I told the friendly nurse, "I am a pain patient," something clearly shifted. The moment I disclosed the name of my prescription medication, her eyes narrowed and judgment filled the space between us.

As the daughter of a physician, I was aware that people often lie to procure pain medicine from emergency-room doctors. Although I never asked for any medication, I understood that my honest response triggered the nurse's doubts about the *real* reason for my visit. She thought I only wanted additional pain medication, and I later learned she passed her suspicions on to the doctor.

When the doctor finally came to examine me, the pain was so intense that I instinctively grabbed her arms when she pressed on my abdomen. I was mortified, but she didn't even flinch. Unaffected and unapologetic, the doctor was hard as nails, undoubtedly also suspecting that my pain wasn't real. Thankfully, she ordered a sonogram anyway. The technician who administered the test was the first person who treated me with kindness. After reading the scan, the doctor who had been so dismissive of my pain entered my room. Compassion—and possibly remorse—filled her eyes as she explained that I needed emergency surgery. I was hemorrhaging internally from a ruptured ovarian cyst. Absurdly, my elation at being believed outweighed my distress about my medical crisis.

The nurse still wore a haughty look when she returned to my

room. Aware that misjudging a patient can lead to a misdiagnosis, I gently asked her, "So, is this the diagnosis you'd expected?" She made no attempt to hide her disdain. "Not necessarily."

She was still treating me with arrogance and contempt. Job must have felt similar despair when he poured out this lament: "My spirit is crushed, and my life is nearly snuffed out. The grave is ready to receive me. I am surrounded by mockers. I watch how bitterly they taunt me. You must defend my innocence, O God, since no one else will stand up for me" (Job 17:1–3, NLT).

Even as I was ebbing away, I wanted to correct her assumptions about me by telling her I was a faith-filled woman who was desperately trying to live with a devastating disease. Graciously, the Lord mediated our unspoken conflict by reminding me to let the peace of Christ rule my heart. In the end, I should not have worried about defending myself, because God had orchestrated a defense even more compelling than the sonogram.

The hospital staff woke an on-call surgeon and told him to rush to the hospital to perform emergency surgery, honestly explaining their mistaken assumption and their surprise upon learning I was actually hemorrhaging. Then they told him my name.

Later recounting this story to me, he said he was so shocked that he asked them to repeat my name and then proclaimed, "I know her! She has a horribly painful disease. Our kids are friends at school, and she goes to my church." They had called the only physician at that hospital who knew me personally. He vigorously defended both my character and the validity of my disabling disease. I was grateful for his support but sobered when he revealed his professional opinion: I would have died if treatment had been delayed any further.

Receiving judgment for our medication choices doesn't typically put our lives in jeopardy, but it will often drive our emotions into turmoil. And our suffering can be compounded by condemnation we receive from others. Beloved, shame is not from God. Condemnation is never part of a prescription for healing.

Are you taking medications you would rather not ingest? Are you embarrassed that you cannot push through your pain without swallowing a pill? We are free to take—or not take—our doctor's prescriptions without being ashamed that our broken bodies require a substance to ease suffering or manage disease. There is no condemnation *ever* for those who are forgiven in Christ Jesus.

Pray: Dear God, please lead me to medications and treatments that enable me to live the life You planned for me. Help me afford my medication without incurring an emotional price because of someone else's judgment. Release me from the side effects of shame and condemnation. Help me forgive those who do not support or understand my medical decisions. Thank You for rising to my defense and delighting in my well-being. You are my peace. In Jesus's name, amen.

Embrace: Shame and condemnation will never be part of my prescription for healing.

Ponder: The apostle Paul instructed Timothy, "Stop drinking only water, and use a little wine because of your stomach and your frequent illnesses" (1 Timothy 5:23). The Greek word for "illnesses" in this verse, *astheneias*, refers to an ailment that robs the sufferer of strength and "*deprives someone* of enjoying or accomplishing what they would like to do."[7] Proper medication usage can restore your ability to function and enjoy your life. How does living with shame for taking those medications steal your strength?

Worship: "No Condemnation" by Anthony Evans

A Glorious View

I remain confident of this: I will see the goodness of the LORD in the land of the living. Wait for the LORD; be strong and take heart and wait for the LORD.

—*Psalm 27:13–14*

I once had to drive on a winding mountain road in severe winter conditions. Since I am from Florida, this took great concentration and patience. I drove my car with a laser-like focus on the road ahead, so I never even noticed the mountains or the beauty around me. After I reached my destination, an awe-inspiring view of the landscape was my reward.

I recently traveled down a long road of physical ailments. Health crisis after health crisis crashed into me, forcing me into the slow lane and often to the side of the road altogether. It is hard to keep going when your body breaks down over and over again. There were times when I wanted to quit trying, but it turns out that this grueling trip has been worth it. I wish everyone could see the glorious view without traveling a similar road, but a steep climb seems to be the only way here. I have a perspective of the landscape of my life that I would never have without my journey through illness. *The view from here is glorious.*

Before illness, I could get out of bed in the morning without making a great effort to move my body. I did not have to use one hand to loosen the spasming clawlike fingers of the other. My regular morning prayers did not include asking God to stop the burning in my body and the bone-crushing pain in my feet. When I was healthy, it was easy to accomplish tasks like showering, getting dressed, and driving my children to school.

I now grieve not only the loss of my former life but also how my health issues have affected my husband and children. There are wholesome meals I did not make, school events I have not attended, and family outings I could not join. But on the rare occasions when medicine and miracle converge to help me function, I revel in the blessing and satisfaction of caring for my family. Feats that before illness were commonplace and—dare I say it?—burdensome are now wondrous accomplishments. Formerly mundane tasks such as going to the store and cooking are a cause for triumphant celebration. *The view from here is glorious.*

Since every activity causes significant pain and fatigue, something is worth doing only when it positively affects those around me. I do not have as much to give anymore, so I must make what I do give count. I have learned that the activities most worth suffering for are the ones that enrich and bless others. The particular people I have a burden to bless are those who are traveling up the same road but are broken down by its side and unable to go on. "Keep going," I want to tell them, "because *the view from here is glorious.*"

The poor and the suffering, the weak and the lost—did these ever settle deeply into my thoughts before? I would have brief moments of concern, but my thoughts and actions were like a butterfly that alights on one flower after another and flits off as quickly as it came. They were of no real consequence. Now I have greater urgency and a burning desire to bless, along with a question in my heart: *What can I do with my gifts despite the limitations I have been given?* So now I pray, "God, show me how I can share the truth of Your vast sufficiency with those who need it the most. Fill me to overflowing with the power of Your Holy Spirit. Let people see Jesus instead of me."

Yes, my daughter, God whispers to me. *Now the view from here is truly glorious.*

Pray: Lord, thank You for guiding me and giving me the strength I need to persevere through difficult parts of my journey. Please send help and repair me when I am broken down and want to give up. Give me faith that sharpens my vision so I can see hope on the road ahead. Open up opportunities to be a blessing to others I meet along the way. Thank You for the perspective to see a glorious view despite the clouds of pain and disease. Amen.

Embrace: Stormy conditions might temporarily cloud my vision, but I will soon be rewarded by a glorious view.

Ponder: What blessings or abilities have you been able to appreciate more since you developed health issues? Describe the glorious view you can see today.

Worship: "God Is Good" by Francesca Battistelli

The Gift That Keeps On Giving

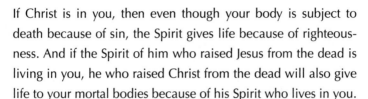

If Christ is in you, then even though your body is subject to death because of sin, the Spirit gives life because of righteousness. And if the Spirit of him who raised Jesus from the dead is living in you, he who raised Christ from the dead will also give life to your mortal bodies because of his Spirit who lives in you.
—*Romans 8:10–11*

Those of us with chronic health issues experience the fragility of life on a daily basis. We feel the brokenness of illness and know that our mortal bodies are not designed to live forever. But we still long to be healthy for as many years as possible. Wouldn't it be wonderful if we could be completely healed and live in a peace-filled world where nothing could harm us? Now imagine living like this for eternity. What a gift that would be! Would you like to receive this gift of restoration? What if I told you that it comes with an unlimited supply of strength, hope, and joy? Are you interested? Then let me tell you how you can receive it.

We know that we are living in a broken world; we see evidence all around us. Watching the evening news is enough to convince us that humans are capable of great wrongdoing. But even the slightest transgression is called sin, and it separates us from the holy and righteous God who created us. The judgment for sin is eternal death. But God loved us so much that He provided us with a wonderful gift that frees us from it. Have you received this gift? It is complete forgiveness of sin and restoration to eternal life through Jesus Christ. God sent His only Son to die on a cross and take the full punishment that our sins deserve. Jesus is the only one able to pay the price for sin, because

He is the only human who never sinned. Jesus, fully God and fully human, took the curse of sin on Himself because He loves us.

If that were the end of the story, it would be a sad story. But it does not end there! God is the Author of life. He brought Jesus back to life three days after He died and was placed in the tomb. Jesus triumphed over death, and He did not do it quietly. He made a spectacle out of it! He appeared to many people, continuing to perform miracles. His friend and disciple John wrote, "Jesus performed many other signs in the presence of his disciples, which are not recorded in this book. But these are written that you may believe that Jesus is the Messiah, the Son of God, and that by believing you may have life in his name" (John 20:30–31).

You receive eternal life when you believe in and follow Jesus. You also receive the Holy Spirit, a helper in this life and a deposit guaranteeing our life to come. Our mortal bodies will not live forever, but the Spirit lives in us and renews us every day. When we die, we will be fully healed and our liberation from sin and decay will be complete. But until that time, we must grow strong in the Spirit so we can overcome the demands and temptations of our flesh.

There will be days when you feel the heaviness of living in this world. Pain and illness are weights that try to crush us back into the dust from which we came. But when we rely on God, nothing can contain the Spirit. This eternal wellspring bursts forth, through the topsoil of weariness and pain, flooding us with unfailing love, effervescent joy, everlasting peace, long-suffering patience, gentle kindness, pure goodness, and confident faithfulness (see Galatians 5:22). What a beautiful gift!

Pray: Dear God, thank You for sending Jesus so I could be forgiven and made new. It gives me great hope to know I will one day be fully healed and alive for eternity. Thank You for choosing me to be Yours. Teach me what it means to live in the Spirit and walk with You every day. Let Your Spirit work within me to transform me. In Jesus's name, amen.

Embrace: I will rely on God and grow strong in the Spirit so I can overcome the demands and temptations of my flesh.

Ponder: Have you accepted the gift of life that Jesus offers? If so, then you already know the assurance that comes from faith. If not, why are you hesitating? If it seems too good to be true, ask God to give you faith to know the truth. He promises, "Call to me and I will answer you and tell you great and unsearchable things you do not know" (Jeremiah 33:3). For more information on how to know Jesus, see page 261.

Worship: "I Have a Savior (Live)" by CeCe Winans

Acknowledgments

Mark: Today I came across a letter you wrote in 2013, when I was bedridden and we thought that was the worst it could get. You wrote, "I am faithfully and fully devoted to you and will always be here to take care of you." And you proved it throughout many more years of my disability, trips to surgical centers, meals on trays, and fancy lunch boxes with little notes for my chemo days. This is not the life we would have chosen or the life we thought we'd have. But His plan was greater than ours. The book you now hold in your hands is a testimony of God's faithfulness to us. He chose you to be my love and the one who makes me laugh the most—even in a hospital room. You have always been the right Mark for me. I love you. P.S. Thank you for understanding that it's best if you do not sing the words of *Incurable Faith* for the audio version. We will just keep your singing gift to ourselves for now.

My Children: Incurable Faith is *your* story too. Thank you for encouraging me to tell it. I'll never forget your helping with my website and social media, or the time when one of you said, "It's okay if you don't make dinner. You are doing something more important," when I was completing my manuscript. "Three things will last forever—faith, hope, and love—and the greatest of these is love" (1 Corinthians 13:13, NLT). I know this is true, because my love for all of you will last forever. Remember that my prayers for you are not confined to a certain time or place; the Lord continues to answer them. I love you!

Dad: The sound of your voice saying, "Write your book!" will never leave me. Perhaps it's because you have been saying it for more than three decades! You prayed for *Incurable Faith* years before I started writing, and then you prayed *with* me—sometimes daily—through every part of this process. You are my biggest champion and cheerleader. Thank you for never giving up on anything or anyone. You leave a legacy of healing that reaches far beyond your sixty years of medical practice. Dad, I love you.

Nan: I love you. A heartfelt thank-you to you and your prayer-warrior friends, whose names I don't know but whose prayers have fueled my ministry to others who suffer. I'm forever grateful that you introduced me to Carolyn Reed Master so I could take the first steps in creating my proposal for *Incurable Faith.* Last, thank you for sharing my writing with your high school friend Maggie, who encourages me daily to keep pressing on.

Elisa and Eric Stanford of Edit Resource: Eric, your thoughtful consideration in choosing editors for *Incurable Faith* led to my dreams becoming a reality. I'll always remember with gratitude the day you stepped in to help and introduced me to Elisa. Elisa, you earned the moniker "Secret Agent" when you followed your instinct to share *Incurable Faith* with Laura. You are a joy to work with, and our friendship has been an unexpected and delightful gift. Thank you for being such a cheerleader for those who are afflicted and need biblical encouragement, support, and love.

Margot Starbuck: People might confuse the ship-captain heritage of the name *Starbuck* with the coffee place, but both reflect your roles in my life. God used your editorial navigation to steer *Incurable Faith* exactly where it needed to go. And your friendship has added a jolt of enlivening humor, warm comfort, and just plain fun to my life. We didn't fulfill our mutual childhood dream of becoming Solid Gold Dancers (yet!), but one day we will dance together on streets of gold.

Multnomah Staff—Laura Barker, Susan Tjaden, Douglas Mann, Brett Benson, Abby DeBenedittis: I am blessed and honored to call Multnomah my publishing home. It has been a privilege to work with all of you. Laura, thank you for seeing the potential for *Incurable Faith* to minister to readers. Susan and Abby, working with you both was a delight! Your thoughtful edits were the final polish the book needed. Douglas and Brett, thank you for your encouragement, dedication, and creativity in promoting *Incurable Faith.*

Don Gates of the Gates Group: Don, thank you for being my agent. Your invaluable advice, wisdom, and prayers helped me navigate this publishing journey.

Sarah Martin and my editors at iBelieve and Crosswalk: Thank you for providing my first opportunity to work as a professional writer. You are an incredible team!

Konni, Marguerite, and Sandy: Sister-friends throughout life no matter what comes our way. I'm grateful for our decades of friendship, prayer, encouragement, and laughter. I love you!

Claire: You have faithfully prayed for me and supported me throughout these difficult decades. I cannot thank you enough for taking me under your wing when your nest was already so full!

The Prayer Warriors (Cori, Jennifer, Julie, Neisha, Sande, Sandy B., Sandy L., and Tammy): You nurtured *Incurable Faith* from conception to birth through your sacrifice of time, prayer, and faith-filled encouragement. You are faithful book doulas! Thank you for being a beautiful part of this miracle.

Abundant Life for Abundant Illness Facebook Group Members: We are fellow travelers in this difficult world of health issues, and I am grateful that our shepherd guides us as we travel together. Thank you for supporting and praying for *Incurable Faith.*

Jen: You are more than an ICU nurse; you are a warrior who fights for people to have the will to live through their toughest health battles. Thank you for arming me with God's truth during my battle. Your nursing skills and exceptional care helped make this book possible.

Kimberlee: Your heart to provide healing care combined with your skillful training has made you a precious part of my life for decades. Thank you for your enthusiastic support thoughout every stage of *Incurable Faith*!

To all my doctors, nurses, and physical therapists: Thank you for your dedication and care. You each have a special place in my heart!

To all the helpers, too numerous to mention, who have come alongside our family: I am grateful for you. Caregiving isn't always the task of one committed person. Sometimes it's an individual answering a temporary calling to help someone who is sick. Thank you to everyone, everywhere, who answers this call.

Jesus, my savior and friend: May others who are hungry for healing taste Your sweetness through this book. "He will deliver the needy who cry out, the afflicted who have no one to help" (Psalm 72:12). My words will never be enough, but one day I will thank You face-to-face for all You have done for us.

Resources

You Can Know Jesus

Trusting Jesus opens the door to spiritual peace. Do you want to . . .

- trade the weight of every wrong for the peace of forgiveness?
- exchange the burden of shame for a renewed spirit?
- extinguish the fear of death with the assurance of eternal life with God?

Our sinful human nature separates us from our perfect and holy creator. The result is death and spiritual separation from God. But He sent His Son to die in our place! Jesus was without sin and died to take the full punishment for our sins. He rose again from the grave, and He offers us the free gift of eternal life. Jesus said, "I am the way and the truth and the life. No one comes to the Father except through me" (John 14:6).

Would you like to know how to trust Jesus so you can be completely forgiven, be made new, and have eternal life?

1. Admit that you need forgiveness and want to find peace with God.
2. Surrender your life to God by believing that Jesus Christ died for you on the cross and rose from the grave.
3. Ask Jesus to forgive your sins and help you follow Him.

Have you decided to follow Jesus? Your next step is to find a local Bible-teaching church to attend. Are you too sick to leave your home? Call the church, and ask if someone there can help you connect with a pastor or other church members. You can find a list of local churches at https://churches.goingfarther.net.

Helpful Scriptures

God's presence *comforts* during lonely seasons:

> The LORD is close to the brokenhearted and saves those who are crushed in spirit. (Psalm 34:18)

> He Himself has said, "I will never leave you nor forsake you." (Hebrews 13:5, NKJV)

> Be strong and courageous. Do not be afraid or terrified because of them, for the LORD your God goes with you; he will never leave you nor forsake you. (Deuteronomy 31:6)

God gives you *courage:*

> Have I not commanded you? Be strong and courageous. Do not be afraid; do not be discouraged, for the LORD your God will be with you wherever you go. (Joshua 1:9)

> Wait for the LORD; be strong and take heart and wait for the LORD. (Psalm 27:14)

> When you pass through the waters, I will be with you; and when you pass through the rivers, they will not sweep over you. When you walk

through the fire, you will not be burned; the flames will not set you ablaze. (Isaiah 43:2)

God helps you *endure* and *persevere:*

We continually ask God to fill you with the knowledge of his will through all the wisdom and understanding that the Spirit gives . . . being strengthened with all power according to his glorious might so that you may have great endurance and patience. (Colossians 1:9, 11)

You need to persevere so that when you have done the will of God, you will receive what he has promised. (Hebrews 10:36)

May the Lord direct your hearts into God's love and Christ's perseverance. (2 Thessalonians 3:5)

God gives you *eternal life:*

The wages of sin is death, but the gift of God is eternal life in Christ Jesus our Lord. (Romans 6:23)

My Father's will is that everyone who looks to the Son and believes in him shall have eternal life, and I will raise them up at the last day. (John 6:40)

God so loved the world that he gave his one and only Son, that whoever believes in him shall not perish but have eternal life. (John 3:16)

God helps you *forgive:*

In him we have redemption through his blood, the forgiveness of sins, in accordance with the riches of God's grace. (Ephesians 1:7)

If you forgive other people when they sin against you, your heavenly Father will also forgive you. But if you do not forgive others their sins, your Father will not forgive your sins. (Matthew 6:14–15)

As God's chosen people, holy and dearly loved, clothe yourselves with compassion, kindness, humility, gentleness and patience. Bear with each other and forgive one another if any of you has a grievance against someone. Forgive as the Lord forgave you. (Colossians 3:12–13)

God gives you *hope:*

May the God of hope fill you with all joy and peace as you trust in him, so that you may overflow with hope by the power of the Holy Spirit. (Romans 15:13)

We also glory in our sufferings, because we know that suffering produces perseverance; perseverance, character; and character, hope. And hope does not put us to shame, because God's love has been poured out into our hearts through the Holy Spirit, who has been given to us. (Romans 5:3–5)

Everything that was written in the past was written to teach us, so that through the endurance taught in the Scriptures and the encouragement they provide we might have hope. (Romans 15:4)

God helps you during *insomnia:*

I lie down and sleep; I wake again, because the LORD sustains me. (Psalm 3:5)

By day the LORD directs his love, at night his song is with me— a prayer to the God of my life. (Psalm 42:8)

In peace I will lie down and sleep, for you alone, LORD, make me dwell in safety. (Psalm 4:8)

God fills you with *joy:*

Restore to me the joy of your salvation and grant me a willing spirit, to sustain me. (Psalm 51:12)

Be joyful in hope, patient in affliction, faithful in prayer. (Romans 12:12)

Rejoice always, pray continually, give thanks in all circumstances; for this is God's will for you in Christ Jesus. (1 Thessalonians 5:16–18)

God gives you *peace:*

You will keep in perfect peace those whose minds are steadfast, because they trust in you. (Isaiah 26:3)

Peace I leave with you; my peace I give you. I do not give to you as the world gives. Do not let your hearts be troubled and do not be afraid. (John 14:27)

Do not be anxious about anything, but in every situation, by prayer and petition, with thanksgiving, present your requests to God. And the peace of God, which transcends all understanding, will guard your hearts and your minds in Christ Jesus. (Philippians 4:6–7)

God always *provides:*

My God will meet all your needs according to the riches of his glory in Christ Jesus. (Philippians 4:19)

If that is how God clothes the grass of the field, which is here today and tomorrow is thrown into the fire, will he not much more clothe you—you of little faith? . . . Therefore do not worry about tomorrow, for tomorrow will worry about itself. Each day has enough trouble of its own. (Matthew 6:30, 34)

God is able to bless you abundantly, so that in all things at all times, having all that you need, you will abound in every good work. (2 Corinthians 9:8)

God *hears* your prayers:

The LORD has heard my cry for mercy; the LORD accepts my prayer. (Psalm 6:9)

I call on you, my God, for you will answer me; turn your ear to me and hear my prayer. (Psalm 17:6)

This is the confidence we have in approaching God: that if we ask anything according to his will, he hears us. And if we know that he hears us—whatever we ask—we know that we have what we asked of him. (1 John 5:14–15)

God *strengthens* you:

Do not fear, for I am with you; do not be dismayed, for I am your God. I will strengthen you and help you; I will uphold you with my righteous right hand. (Isaiah 41:10)

We do not lose heart. Though outwardly we are wasting away, yet inwardly we are being renewed day by day. (2 Corinthians 4:16)

If anyone serves, they should do so with the strength God provides, so that in all things God may be praised through Jesus Christ. (1 Peter 4:11)

God helps you withstand *temptation:*

Because he himself suffered when he was tempted, he is able to help those who are being tempted. (Hebrews 2:18)

Submit yourselves, then, to God. Resist the devil, and he will flee from you. (James 4:7)

No temptation has overtaken you except what is common to mankind. And God is faithful; he will not let you be tempted beyond what you can bear. But when you are tempted, he will also provide a way out so that you can endure it. (1 Corinthians 10:13)

God helps you conquer *worry:*

Cast all your anxiety on him because he cares for you. (1 Peter 5:7)

Why, my soul, are you downcast? Why so disturbed within me? Put your hope in God, for I will yet praise him, my Savior and my God. (Psalm 43:5)

Look at the birds of the air; they do not sow or reap or store away in barns, and yet your heavenly Father feeds them. Are you not much more valuable than they? Can any one of you by worrying add a single hour to your life? (Matthew 6:26–27)

Further Reading

Alsup, Wendy. *Companions in Suffering: Comfort for Times of Loss and Loneliness.* Downers Grove, Ill.: InterVarsity, 2020.

Butler, Kathryn. *Glimmers of Grace: A Doctor's Reflections on Faith, Suffering, and the Goodness of God.* Wheaton, Ill.: Crossway, 2021.

Carmichael, Amy. *Rose from Brier: A Priceless Treasury of Helpful Thoughts for Those Who Are Ill.* Fort Washington, Pa.: CLC Publications, 2010.

Elliot, Elisabeth. *Suffering Is Never for Nothing.* Nashville: B&H, 2019.

Furman, Dave. *Kiss the Wave: Embracing God in Your Trials.* Wheaton, Ill.: Crossway, 2018.

Lotz, Anne Graham. *Jesus in Me: Experiencing the Holy Spirit as a Constant Companion.* Colorado Springs, Colo.: Multnomah, 2019.

Risner, Vaneetha Rendall. *The Scars That Have Shaped Me: How God Meets Us in Suffering.* Minneapolis: CreateSpace, 2016.

Sala, Harold J. *What You Need to Know About Healing: A Physical and Spiritual Guide.* Nashville: B&H, 2013.

Tada, Joni Eareckson. *A Lifetime of Wisdom: Embracing the Way God Heals You.* Grand Rapids, Mich.: Zondervan, 2009.

Wolf, Katherine, and Jay Wolf. *Suffer Strong: How to Survive Anything by Redefining Everything.* Grand Rapids, Mich.: Zondervan, 2020.

Wolgemuth, Nancy DeMoss, and Robert Wolgemuth. *You Can Trust God to Write Your Story: Embracing the Mysteries of Providence.* Chicago: Moody, 2019.

Yancey, Philip. *Where Is God When It Hurts?* Grand Rapids, Mich.: Zondervan, 1990.

Where to Find Help

If you need mental health support, please seek a referral to a therapist from your physician. Your church should also have a recommended list of therapists.

National Suicide Prevention Lifeline
Dial 988 or 1-800-273-TALK (8255)
Counselors are available 24/7 to support those in distress.

National Hopeline Network, Suicide, and Crisis Hotline
1-800-442-HOPE (4673)
Counselors are available 24/7 to help.

Christian Resources

Celebrate Recovery
A Christ-centered twelve-step recovery program with support groups worldwide. For more information, visit their website: www.celebraterecovery.com

Focus on the Family's Counseling Department
Call 1-855-771-HELP (4357) weekdays from 6:00 A.M. to 8:00 P.M. (MST) for a free counseling consultation and referral with a licensed or pastoral counselor.

Joni and Friends International Disability Center
Joni and Friends is for everyone. They bring "the Gospel and practical resources to people impacted by disability around the globe."[1] From training and programs to outreaches and mentoring, this ministry has something for everyone. I highly encourage you to

look on their website at www.joniandfriends.org or call or text 1-818-707-5664.

Physical Address:	Mailing Address:
30009 Ladyface Court	PO Box 3333
Agoura Hills, CA 91301	Agoura Hills, CA 91376-3333

HIS Radio 24/7 Prayer Line

Call or text 1-866-987-PRAY (7729), or go online at www.hisradio .com.

Caregiver Resources

Christian Caregiver

www.christiancaregiversupport.com (support groups, devotions, and other resources)

Stephen Ministries

www.stephenministries.org (lay congregation members trained to provide one-to-one care to those experiencing difficulties such as grief or chronic or terminal illness)

Author Website

www.andreaherzer.com (resources for caregivers)

Suggested Reading

Brown, Jill Case. *We're Stronger Than We Look: Insights and Encouragement for the Caregiver's Journey.* Colorado Springs, Colo.: NavPress, 2022.

Daly, Jane. *The Caregiving Season: Finding Grace to Honor Your Aging Parents.* Carol Stream, Ill.: Tyndale, 2016.

Rosenberger, Peter. *Hope for the Caregiver.* Brentwood, Tenn.: Worthy Inspired, 2014.

Notes

Section One

1. Taken from Andrea Herzer, "A Prayer for the Peace of Christ—Your Daily Prayer—August 24," Crosswalk.com, August 24, 2021, www .crosswalk.com/devotionals/your-daily-prayer/your-daily-prayer -august-24.html. Used by permission.

2. Taken from Andrea Herzer, "5 Truths That Turn the Tables on Illness," iBelieve, September 10, 2019, www.ibelieve.com/faith/5 -truths-that-turn-the-tables-on-illness.html. Used by permission.

3. Taken from Andrea Herzer, "5 Truths That Turn the Tables on Illness," iBelieve, September 10, 2019, www.ibelieve.com/faith/5 -truths-that-turn-the-tables-on-illness.html. Used by permission.

Section Two

1. L. B. Cowman, *Streams in the Desert: 366 Daily Devotional Readings* (Grand Rapids, Mich.: Zondervan, 1997), 147.

2. Jennifer Rothschild, *Lessons I Learned in the Dark: Steps to Walking by Faith, Not by Sight* (Colorado Springs, Colo.: Multnomah, 2002), 207.

3. Steven E. Mock and Susan M. Arai, "Childhood Trauma and Chronic Illness in Adulthood: Mental Health and Socioeconomic Status as Explanatory Factors and Buffers," *Frontiers in Psychology* 1, no. 246 (January 31, 2011), doi:10.3389/fpsyg.2010.00246.

4. Taken from Andrea Herzer, "5 Truths That Turn the Tables on Illness," iBelieve, September 10, 2019, www.ibelieve.com/faith/5-truths-that-turn-the-tables-on-illness.html. Used by permission.

5. Matthew Henry, *Matthew Henry Commentary* (Grand Rapids, Mich.: Zondervan, 1960), 1264.

6. François de Salignac de La Mothe-Fénelon, quoted in Mary W. Tileston, ed., *Joy and Strength for the Pilgrim's Day* (Boston: Little, Brown, 1909), 82.

7. Charles Stanley, *I Lift Up My Soul: Devotions to Start Your Day with God* (Nashville: Thomas Nelson, 2010), 29.

Section Three

1. Lucy C. Smith, quoted in Tileston, *Joy and Strength,* 237.

2. Amy Carmichael, *Rose from Brier: A Priceless Treasury of Helpful Thoughts for Those Who Are Ill* (Fort Washington, Pa.: CLC Publications, 2010), 105.

3. Georg Neumark, quoted in Tileston, *Joy and Strength,* 292.

4. Henri J. M. Nouwen, *Reaching Out: The Three Movements of the Spiritual Life* (New York: Bantam, Dell, Doubleday, 1986), 34.

5. Os Hillman, *TGIF: Today God Is First; Daily Workplace Inspiration* (Ventura, Calif.: Regal, 2007), 2:90.

6. John Piper, *Lessons from a Hospital Bed* (Wheaton, Ill.: Crossway, 2016), 52–53.

7. "769. Astheneia," Bible Hub, https://biblehub.com/greek/769.htm.

Resources

1. "What We Do," Joni and Friends, www.joniandfriends.org/about/what-we-do.

Topical Index

The following list will help you find a devotion according to your need. Some devotions are included in multiple categories. Topics listed are not exhaustive.